BRITISH COLUMBIA CANCER AGENCY
LIBRARY
600 W
VANC
V5Z 4E6
D0154346

This publication was sponsored by ICI Pharmaceuticals.
The pharmaceuticals business of ICI PLC has now been transferred to Zeneca Limited.

BRITISH COLUMBIA CANCER AGENCY
LIBRARY
600 WEST 10th AVE.
VANCOUVER, B.C. CANADA
V5Z 4E6

Uterine Fibroids

Time for Review

Advances
in Reproductive
Endocrinology

VOLUME 4

Uterine Fibroids

Time for Review

Edited by RW Shaw

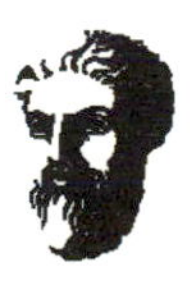

The Parthenon Publishing Group
International Publishers in Medicine, Science & Technology

**Casterton Hall, Carnforth,
Lancs, LA6 2LA, UK**

**120 Mill Road, Park Ridge,
New Jersey 07656, USA**

Published in the UK by
The Parthenon Publishing Group Limited
Casterton Hall, Carnforth,
Lancs, LA6 2LA, England

Published in the USA by
The Parthenon Publishing Group Inc.
120 Mill Road,
Park Ridge,
New Jersey 07656, USA

Copyright © 1992 Parthenon Publishing Group Ltd

British Library Cataloguing in Publication Data
Uterine Fibroids: Time for Review. –
(Advances in Reproductive Endocrinology
Series; v. 4)
I. Shaw, Robert W. II. Series
618.1

ISBN 1-85070-430-9

Library of Congress Cataloging-in-Publication Data
Uterine fibroids : time for review / edited by R.W. Shaw
p. cm. — (Advances in reproductive endocrinology : v. 4)
Includes bibliographical references and index.
ISBN 1-85070-430-9
1. Uterine fibroids — Congresses. I. Shaw, Robert W. (Robert Wayne) II. Series
[DNLM: 1. Leiomyoma — etiology — congresses. 2. Leiomyoma — pathology — congresses. 3. Uterine Neoplasms — etiology — congresses. 4. Uterine Neoplasm — pathology — congresses. W1 AD83S v. 4 / WP 459 U89]
RC280.U8U74 1992
616.99'266—dc20
DNLM/DLC
for Library of Congress 92-12154
CIP

No part of this book may be reproduced in any form without permission from the publishers except for the quotation of brief passages for the purposes of review

Composition by Ryburn Typesetting Ltd, Halifax, England
Printed and bound in Great Britain by
Butler and Tanner, Frome and London

Contents

List of principal contributors

D.H. Barlow
Nuffield Department of Obstetrics and Gynaecology
John Radcliffe Hospital
Maternity Department
Headington
Oxford OX3 9DU
UK

J. Crow
Histopathology Department
Royal Free Hospital School of Medicine
Rowland Hill Street
London NW3
UK

J. Donnez
Department of Gynecology
Cliniques Universitaires Saint-Luc
ASBL
Avenue Hippocrate 10
B-1200 Brussels
Belgium

R.L. Gardner
Academic Department of Obstetrics and Gynaecology
Royal Free Hospital School of Medicine
Pond Street
London NW3 2QG
UK

A. Gordon
Consultant Obstetrician and Gynaecologist
Princess Royal Maternity Hospital
Hedon Road
Hull
UK

M.A. Lumsden
Simpson Memorial Maternity Pavilion
Royal Infirmary of Edinburgh
Lauriston Place
Edinburgh EH3 9EF
UK

G. McSweeney
Academic Department of Obstetrics and Gynaecology
Royal Free Hospital and School of Medicine
Pond Street
London NW3 2QG
UK

R. Maheux
Endocrinology of Reproduction Department
Hospital St. Francois d'Assisi
10 Rue de l'Espinay
Quebec
Canada

K.-W. Schweppe
Department of Obstetrics and Gynaecology
Academic Teaching Hospital of the University of Göttingen
Lange Straße 38
D-2910 Westerstede
Germany

R.W. Shaw
Academic Department of Obstetrics and Gynaecology
Royal Free Hospital and School of Medicine
Pond Street
London NW3 2QG
UK

E.J. Thomas
Department of Human Reproduction and Obstetrics
The Princess Anne Hospital
Coxford Road
Southampton SO9 4HA
UK

P. Vercellini
Department of Obstetrics and Gynaecology
Ia Clinica Obstetica e Ginecologica
Via Commenda 12
20122 Milano
Italy

C.P. West
Department of Obstetrics and Gynaecology
Royal Infirmary
Lauriston Place
Edinburgh EH3 9YW
UK

Foreword

Uterine fibroids (leiomyomas) are one of the commonest benign tumours to affect the female reproductive organs and are often an indication for performing hysterectomy. How much do we understand of their aetiology and pathology, and what symptoms are really attributable to their presence? These basic questions need to be answered adequately before we can judge whether current treatment options are appropriate and were some of those addressed during our third International Workshop in Reproductive Endocrinology, held at the Gleneagles Hotel, in October 1991. The meeting was kindly sponsored by ICI Pharmaceuticals (UK) and brought together a group of interested clinicians and researchers.

The above questions were amongst many issues debated and our apparent lack of knowledge in these fundamental areas in relation to fibroids became obvious. The development of new endoscopic equipment, particularly laparoscopic laser options and hysteroscopic surgical techniques, have opened up new and less invasive surgical procedures for many patients. Many of these endoscopic approaches rely not only upon appropriate selection but also on medical preparation, and here the role and value of gonadotropin releasing hormone (GnRH) analogues became apparent.

Whilst, then, we have achieved significant advances in the medical and surgical treatment options for uterine fibroids, further advances must await our continued research into the basic aspects of initiation and growth of these ubiquitous tumours, to try and develop methods of prevention.

Professor Robert W. Shaw
Academic Department of Obstetrics and Gynaecology
Royal Free Hospital and School of Medicine
London

1

The aetiology and pathogenesis of fibroids

E.J. Thomas

INTRODUCTION

Fibroids are benign neoplasms of the uterine smooth muscle which are present in between 25 and 30% of all women. They are the commonest tumours in women and account for significant gynaecological morbidity. This paper analyses current knowledge of their aetiology, pathogenesis and complications. It also considers whether there are factors which may influence whether a fibroid becomes malignant.

AETIOLOGY

Fibroids occur virtually exclusively during the reproductive era and regress after the menopause. This strongly suggests that they are oestrogen dependent, and this has been verified recently by the observation that they shrink when a hypo-oestrogenic state is induced with gonadotropin releasing hormone (GnRH) agonist therapy[1]. There is a racial bias in the development of these tumours, as they are up to nine times more common in Negroes than Caucasians. There is also a genetic tendency towards fibroids, with first order relatives of sufferers more likely to have them[2]. The combination of both the racial and genetic tendencies suggests that this predisposition is a result of differing gene expression rather than environmental factors. Thus far, no gene has been described that is expressed more commonly in women with fibroids.

It is logical to hypothesize that factors which alter endogenous oestrogen secretion will alter the incidence of fibroids, because they are oestrogen-dependent tumours. Fibroids are commoner in obese women who show a high conversion of androgens to oestrogens in peripheral adipose tissue. They have a lower incidence in women who take an oral contraceptive and also in those who smoke cigarettes[3]. Although the oral contraceptive induces an oestrogenic state, it is constant and because follicular growth is suppressed, the normal peak plasma concentrations of oestradiol do not occur. Presumably it is these peak plasma concentrations of oestradiol which are important in stimulating fibroid growth. The requirement for high plasma oestradiol concentrations is further supported by the fact that the recurrence or persistence of fibroids is not a major problem in postmenopausal hormone replacement therapy. Cigarette smoking is known to be potently anti-oestrogenic and is associated with a lower incidence of oestrogen-dependent disease such as breast carcinoma and endometriosis[4]. The precise mechanisms for this are unclear but it is known that smoking may suppress follicular oestradiol secretion or alter oestrogen metabolism.

There is an inverse risk of fibroids with increasing parity[1]. Two possible explanations can be forwarded for this. The first is that exposure to oestradiol secretion is interrupted by pregnancies and therefore stimulation to growth is less. The fact that pregnancy itself is an oestrogenic state might invalidate this explanation, and clinicians are well aware that changes can occur to fibroids during pregnancy. However, the principal oestrogen in pregnancy is not oestradiol and it may be that it is this steroid in particular which stimulates fibroid growth. The alternative explanation is that there is mechanical disruption to the uterine musculature as a result of the stretching that occurs during pregnancy and that this decreases the risk of fibroids.

PATHOGENESIS

Macroscopic and microscopic features

Fibroids contain both smooth muscle fibres and connective tissue. They also contain vascular lakes and changes in blood flow occur through the uterine artery[1,5]. The fibroids originate from one muscle cell, as demonstrated by the fact that they show consistency in electrophoretic patterns of the enzyme glucose-6-phosphate dehydrogenase[6]. These electrophoretic patterns are characteristic for each particular cell such that a tumour of polyclonal origin will show varied patterns whereas one of monoclonal origin will express a single pattern. Each fibroid originates from a specific muscle cell and is not a metastasis of a primary tumour.

Macroscopically, fibroids are well-demarcated tumours which show a characteristic whorled appearance. They can be single or multiple and can vary in size from very small tumours to growths that fill the whole abdomen. They can occur in any part of the uterine musculature, and in the cervix and are named by their specific position in the uterus as either subserosal, intramural or submucous. They can also become pedunculated, and if this occurs in a submucous fibroid it can appear through the cervix and is termed a fibroid polyp. Very occasionally, a pedunculated sub-serosal fibroid becomes detached from the uterus and attaches to adjacent structures within the abdomen; this is termed a parasitic fibroid.

Cellular mechanisms of pathogenesis

The precise mechanisms that stimulate the abnormal growth of the single uterine smooth muscle cell are unknown. As discussed above there is considerable circumstantial evidence which suggests that endogenous oestrogen stimulation is important. There is also recent evidence that growth factors, especially epidermal growth factor, play a major role in the pathogenesis of fibroids[7]. These are discussed in detail in Chapter 2 by Dr Lumsden, and therefore this paper will concentrate on the ovarian steroids. However, there is now considerable evidence that the ovarian steroids exert their effect through the paracrine influence of growth factors, as well as through gene transcription mediated through their receptors. Growth factors will also influence the expression of steroid receptors and so the effects of steroids and growth factors are interdependent and any separation is artificial.

A muscle cell may grow abnormally in response to an oestrogenic signal if either the signal is abnormal or the cell has an increased sensitivity to the signal. The higher incidence of fibroids in obese women provides *in vivo* evidence that an abnormal signal will stimulate growth. However, there appear to have been no published studies that have compared the endocrinology of the menstrual cycle of women with fibroids and those without to determine whether there are increased oestradiol concentrations in the index group. One can speculate that a difference is unlikely to be demonstrated either because of the methodological difficulties or because such a mechanism is biologically simplistic.

The major mechanism by which a cell could become more sensitive to oestrogen would be by altered expression of receptors to the steroids. Various studies have investigated the expression of oestrogen receptors in fibroids. Buchi and Keller[8] could not demonstrate any difference between the expression of oestrogen receptors in the fibroids and in the surrounding myometrium. However, Wilson and colleagues[9], Tamaya and co-workers[10] and Soules and McCarty[11] were able to show different expression in the fibroids compared with the surrounding myometrium and the endometrium. It has also been reported that the expression of both oestrogen and progesterone receptors follows the cyclical pattern in fibroids that is shown in both normal myometrium and endometrium. One study has shown an increased expression of progesterone receptors in fibroids compared to the myometrium in Black women[12]. There is therefore conflicting evidence about the expression of oestrogen and progesterone receptors in fibroids.

These conflicting results can be explained in two ways. Firstly, the control of oestrogen and progesterone receptor expression is complex and depends upon the degree of differentiation of the cell, paracrine influences such as growth factors and the endocrine influence of both the steroids themselves. In view of this multifactorial control it is unlikely that oestrogen and progesterone receptor expression alone could be the only explanation for fibroid growth. Secondly, the methodology for measuring receptor expression is still imprecise and significant confounding variables are evident between the studies.

The use of techniques to measure mRNA transcription for oestrogen and progesterone receptors will provide more insight as to whether there are differences between the control mechanisms in fibroids and in normal myometrium. Further investigations of cellular dysfunction in fibroids could be performed using an *in vitro* model with established cell culture. Hopefully, the use of such techniques in the future will elucidate the relationship between the genetic, endocrine and paracrine factors in the pathogenesis of fibroids.

COMPLICATIONS OF FIBROIDS

Benign

Fibroids can undergo a number of benign changes. They may calcify and also undergo cystic and hyaline degeneration. They can also undergo 'red degeneration' which is typified by a clinical picture of pain and uterine tenderness. Macroscopically, the fibroid appears red and soft and microscopically there are signs of oedema, haemorrhage and necrosis. This occurs most commonly in pregnancy and is thought to be a reflection of the high plasma progesterone concentrations found in that condition. Pedunculated fibroids may also twist on the pedicle and undergo necrosis. There are no satisfactory studies which have explored the factors which may predispose a particular fibroid or individual to degenerative complications of fibroids. Although there is an anecdotal belief that the larger the size of the fibroid, the more likely it is to undergo degeneration, there are no studies to confirm this. Apart from a pedunculated fibroid, no study has shown that the position of a fibroid influences the chances of complications.

Malignant

One of the most persistent debates in gynaecology is whether a fibroid should be removed if it is found by chance and is not causing any symptoms. Benign complications of a fibroid will demonstrate themselves symptomatically and can be dealt with if and when they appear. It may be better to remove a fibroid before pregnancy in order to minimize any complications, although the benefits of this would have to be weighed against the possibilities of tubal damage as a result of the surgery. Essentially, the only reason for removing an asymptomatic fibroid, especially in a woman not requiring future fertility, would be the danger of it becoming malignant.

Leiomyosarcoma is the malignancy associated with fibroids. Histological changes suggesting a leiomyosarcoma are found in 0.1–0.5% of fibroids removed surgically. The peak incidence for leiomyosarcoma is in the sixth decade and after the menopause[1]. This peak is approximately 20 years after that for the fibroids themselves. Because of the rarity of a leiomyosarcoma and the differences in the age of peak incidence, it is impossible to prove that the malignant change has arisen in a fibroid. It is equally likely that it is a *de novo* malignant transformation of a uterine muscle cell. Longitudinal studies showing that benign fibroids can become malignant do not exist. Similarly, there are no studies which have identified factors that may predispose an individual to leiomyosarcoma. In particular there are no studies demonstrating a greater risk of leiomyosarcoma if large fibroids are present.

In view of the paucity of data and the morbidity and mortality of abdominal surgery, there appears to be no justification for treating an asymptomatic fibroid, whatever the size, because it may become malignant. Surgery would appear to be justified only if symptoms appear or abnormalities are detected by ultrasonography.

CONCLUSION

There are genetic and racial tendencies for fibroids. Endogenous and exogenous oestrogens can influence the appearance of fibroids. Ovarian steroids are clearly implicated in their pathogenesis although whether this is mediated as an endocrine or paracrine event by growth factors is unknown. The role of steroid receptors is unclear. Fibroids can undergo benign complications but it is unclear whether this is a malignant transformation or a *de novo* event. Our current knowledge of the natural history of fibroids would suggest that there is little, if any, benefit in prophylactic treatment if the tumour is asymptomatic. The use of molecular biological techniques and the establishment of an *in vitro* model will help to elucidate the pathogenesis of these common tumours.

REFERENCES

1. Lumsden, M.A., West, C.P. and Baird, D.T. (1987). Goserelin therapy before surgery for fibroids. *Lancet*, **1**, 36–7
2. Vollenhoven, B.J., Lawrence, A.S. and Healy, D.L. (1990). Uterine fibroids: a clinical review. *Br. J. Obstet. Gynaecol.*, **97**, 285–98
3. Ross, P.K., Pike, M.C., Vessey, M.P., Bull, D., Yeates, D. and Casagrande, J.T. (1986). Risk factors for uterine fibroids: reduced risk

associated with oral contraceptives. *Br. Med. J.*, **293**, 359–63

4. Goldman, M.B. and Cramer, D.W. (1990). The epidemiology of endometriosis. In Chadha, D.R. and Buttram, V.C. (eds.) *Current Concepts in Endometriosis.* (New York: Alan R. Liss)
5. Matta, W.M.H., Stabile, I., Shaw, R.W. and Campbell, S. (1988). Doppler assessment of uterine blood flow changes in patients with fibroids receiving the gonadotrophin releasing hormone agonist buserelin. *Fertil. Steril.*, **46**, 1083–5
6. Townsend, D.E., Sparkes, R.S., Baluda, M.C. and McCelland, G. (1970). Unicellular histogenesis of uterine leiomyomas as determined by electrophoresis of glucose-6-phosphate dehydrogenase. *Am. J. Obstet. Gynecol.*, **107**, 1168–74
7. Lumsden, M.A., West, C.P., Bromley, J., Rumgay, L. and Baird, D.T. (1988). The binding of epidermal growth factor to the human uterus and leiomyomata in women rendered hypo-oestrogenic by continuous administration of an LHRH-agonist. *Br. J. Obstet. Gynaecol.*, **95**, 1299–1304
8. Buchi, K.A. and Keller, P.J. (1980). Estrogen receptors in normal and myomatous human uteri. *Gynecol. Obstet. Invest.*, **11**, 59–60
9. Wilson, E.A., Yang, F. and Rees, D. (1980). Estradiol and progesterone binding in uterine leiomyomata and normal uterine tissues. *Obstet. Gynecol.*, **55**, 20–3
10. Tamaya, T., Fujimoto, J. and Okada, H. (1985). Comparison of cellular levels of steroid receptors in uterine leiomyomata and endometrium. *Acta Obstet. Gynecol. Scand.*, **64**, 307–9
11. Soules, M.R. and McCarty, K.S. (1982). Leiomyomas steroid receptor content. *Am. J. Obstet. Gynecol.*, **143**, 6–11
12. Sadan, O., Vaniddekinge, B., Van Gelderen, C.J., Savage, N., Becker, P.J., Van Der Walt, L.A. and Robinson, M. (1987). Oestrogen and progesterone receptor concentrations in leiomyoma and normal myometrium. *Ann. Clin. Biochem.*, **24**, 263–7

2

The role of oestrogen and growth factors in the control of the growth of uterine leiomyomata

M.A. Lumsden

THE MECHANISM OF ACTION OF OESTROGEN

Steroids exert their effects after combining with receptors. Receptors are present within the nucleus although combination with hormone occurs in the cytoplasm, possibly as part of a recycling mechanism. The theory that unoccupied receptors are present in the cytoplasm and occupied in the nucleus is no longer thought to be accurate[1]. The oestrogen–receptor complex acts as a transcription factor and is important in regulating expression of specific genes. Oestrogen binding controls at least two distinct steps in receptor activation: firstly it promotes receptor dimerization and high affinity DNA binding; secondly it induces full transcriptional activity of the receptor[2]. After combination with DNA it affects production of oestrogen-dependent proteins by altering production of the messenger RNA (mRNA). All oestrogen-responsive tissues have receptors, although not all the cells within such tissues will contain them. This may be due to heterogeneity and may also account for the variable response of the tissues to hormonal stimulation. Oestrogen-sensitive tissues include uterus, breast and connective tissues such as skin and bone. However, how oestrogen actually exerts it effects within these tissues is not completely clear. One possibility is that production of local factors may affect neighbouring cells (autocrine) or those further afield (paracrine).

Oestrogen and the uterus

Oestrogen is known to have a trophic effect on both normal myometrium and uterine fibroids. Fibroids never occur before puberty and also shrink after the menopause. The gonadotropin hormone releasing hormone agonists induce a hypo-oestrogenic state which is accompanied by fibroid shrinkage[3,4]. Steroid receptors have been demonstrated in both fibroid and myometrium[5–7] and binding occurs to a vast majority of fibroids, but fails to occur in around one in twenty cases. This may be due to the cellular composition or to other unknown factors. It is thought that binding to the fibroid is greater than to the myometrium in many cases. Farber and colleagues[5] demonstrated a 20% greater uptake of oestradiol by fibroid tissue in seven out of ten cases, but did not feel that decreased binding was associated with an unresponsive fibroid. Puukka and colleagues[6] also found a greater binding to fibroid homogenates (fibroid, mean ± SD: 98 ± 108 fmol/mg cytosol protein) compared to a figure of 79 ± 69 for myometrium although the difference failed to reach statistical significance. These findings are also supported by the studies of Wilson and colleagues[7] and Lumsden and co-workers[8]. However, some workers have failed to show a difference between the two tissue types[9,10]. This may be due either to differences in methodology or to an insufficient number of tumours examined.

The influence of steroids on receptor levels

Oestradiol is known to stimulate the formation of its own receptor, with highest concentrations occurring in the follicular and peri-ovulatory phases[11,12]. Levels then decline in the secretory phase, possibly because of the effects of progesterone. However, there is no correlation between either serum or tissue levels of oestrogen and oestrogen binding in normally cycling women[6,8,12] and there is also no relationship between the circulating oestradiol concentration and the presence of fibroids[13]. Thus it is unlikely that oestrogen is the only important factor.

THE GONADOTROPIN HORMONE-RELEASING HORMONE AGONISTS

If fibroid growth is under the control of oestrogen alone then a decrease in fibroid size might be expected to be accompanied by a decrease in oestradiol binding. The GnRH agonists induce a decrease in fibroid size which is thought to be a result of the hypo-oestrogenic state induced by these drugs as a result of pituitary down-regulation[3,4]. An alternative explanation would be a direct action of the agonist on the fibroid itself. Although specific binding of GnRH agonist has been demonstrated[14], we have been unable to confirm these results (M.A. Lumsden and T. Bramley, unpublished observations). Any effect is likely to be unimportant clinically since the agonists have no effect on fibroid size in postmenopausal women (M.A. Lumsden and C.P. West, unpublished observations). Therefore, the decrease in circulating oestradiol is the most likely cause of fibroid shrinkage and we have therefore studied the relationship between the latter and the concentration of oestradiol receptors. The concentrations of both unoccupied and total receptor populations were measured. Unoccupied receptor content is measured by incubating tissue homogenate with radiolabelled hormone and then separating the bound from the free hormone using dextran-coated charcoal (Figure 1). 'Total' receptor concentration was measured using a double monoclonal antibody technique. The measurement of total receptor concentration is important since occupancy of receptors varies during the menstrual cycle according to the circulating level of oestradiol. Oestradiol receptor concentration was measured in fibroid and myometrium collected from normally cycling women and those pretreated with the GnRH agonist Zoladex®. We were surprised to find that the binding of oestradiol was significantly greater in the agonist-treated women[8] (Figure 2). However, a precedent for our findings has been set by work on pre- and postmenopausal women with breast cancer[15] and in whole human uterus[12] where greater concentrations were found in tissues from postmenopausal patients. One possible explanation is that the occupancy of oestradiol receptors in postmenopausal and agonist-treated women is very low because of the low circulating oestradiol levels. However, total oestradiol receptor levels in tissues from agonist-treated women measured by enzymeimmunoassay (EIA) do not differ significantly from that measured by dextran-coated charcoal (DCC) assay (Figure 2). The findings are consistent with

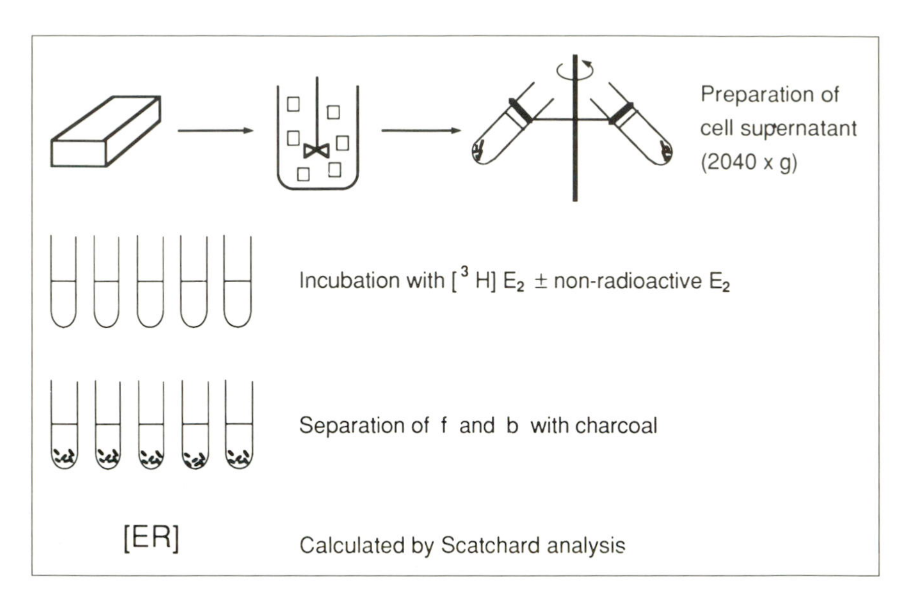

Figure 1 The method employed to measure unoccupied oestrogen receptor (ER) content. Tissue preparation involves weighing, homogenization and centrifugation. The incubation step involves dispensing of cytosol into pre-prepared tubes of 'hot' + 'cold' oestradiol (E_2), including an 'excess oestrogen' tube to assess non-specific binding. After overnight incubation, charcoal suspension is added then centrifuged and the supernatant counted. (f = free; b = bound)

experience in breast cancer specimens from postmenopausal women[16] where DCC assay and EIA yield comparable values. In premenopausal patients, however, concentrations measured by EIA exceed those measured by DCC assay[16–18]. Our results support this, in part, since the oestradiol receptor concentrations as measured by the two methods in fibroid biopsies from normally cycling women showed a similar pattern. Also, oestradiol receptor occupancy appears to be small, even in normally cycling women at midcycle, as originally suggested by Sakai and Saez[19]. Since the same rise is observed using the two different assays and since there was no change in affinity, there must be either an increase in synthesis or a decrease in breakdown of oestradiol receptors.

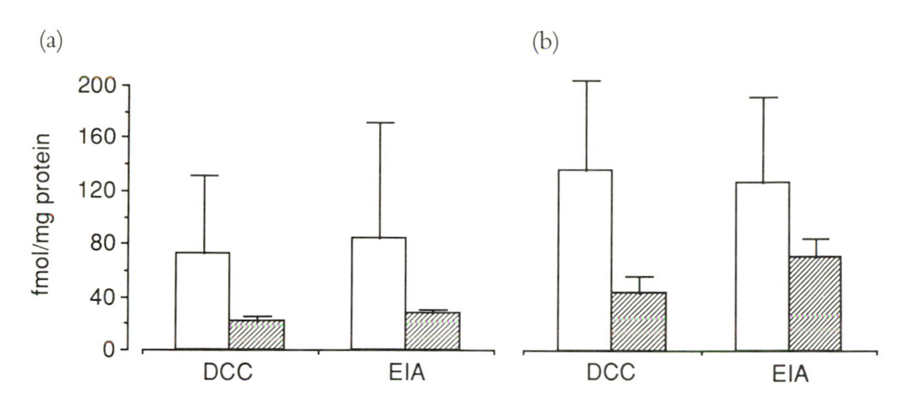

Figure 2 The binding of oestrogen to (a) myometrium and (b) fibroid in women treated with GnRH agonist (clear bars) compared with normal controls (hatched bars), using dextran-coated charcoal (DCC) assay and enzyme immunoassay (EIA)

The action of tamoxifen

In women treated with tamoxifen the 'total' oestradiol receptor concentration in fibroids was significantly less than in normally cycling women (Figure 3). This is likely to be due to the elevated levels of progesterone which are known to be present when tamoxifen is administered continuously[20], therefore raising the possibility that the rise in oestradiol receptors occurring with GnRH agonist is a result of decreased progesterone levels.

THE ROLE OF PROGESTERONE

Attention has been given largely to the effect of oestrogen on fibroid growth, and progesterone has been less extensively studied. Progesterone receptor (PR) concentration shows a pattern similar to that of oestrogen receptor (ER)[8,11,21] indicating that oestradiol stimulates and progesterone inhibits production. PRs are present in both myometrium and fibroid[7,8] in significantly higher concentrations than the oestrogen receptor (Table 1). The PR content is significantly higher in fibroid than in myometrium collected from normally cycling women and is significantly decreased in fibroid biopsies from agonist-treated women[8]. Interestingly,

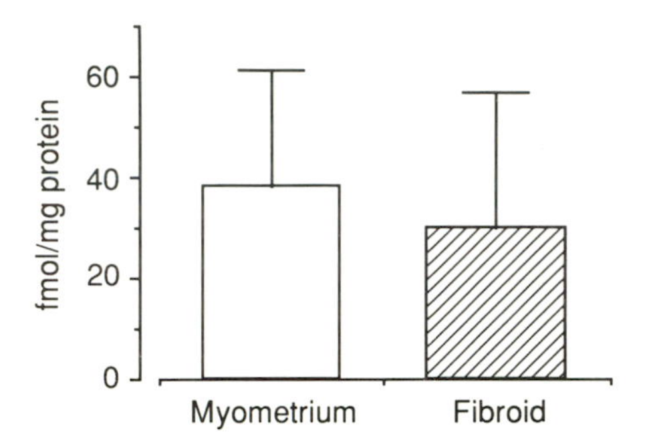

Figure 3 The binding of oestrogen to fibroid and myometrium collected from women treated preoperatively with tamoxifen. This figure shows the receptor content as measured by enzyme immunoassay

Table 1 The effect of GnRH agonist on the concentration of progesterone receptors in the human uterus

	Progesterone receptor (fmol/mg protein)	
	Median	*Range*
Fibroid		
none	531	69–3315
GnRH-a	200	65–1218
Myometrium		
none	250	51–1225
GnRH-a	170	51–723

progesterone receptor may be present even in the absence of ER in about 12% of uteri[12], suggesting that there may be a type of receptor which is independent of oestrogen. Although this did not occur in our study, this may have resulted because our study used myometrium from uteri containing fibroids rather than tissue from normal uteri. The same study[12] also failed to demonstrate a linear relationship between oestrogen and progesterone receptors in the same uterus from normally cycling women, and only one out of the 319 uteri examined was ER- and PR-negative.

There is an inverse relationship between circulating oestradiol and tissue levels of progesterone receptor in the secretory phase[22] and in our study of agonist-treated women a relationship was demonstrated between these levels and mean fibroid size ($r = 0.83$, $p < 0.001$) as well as the binding of progesterone to both fibroid ($r = 0.72$, $p < 0.01$) and myometrium ($r = 0.91$, $p < 0.01$) using Spearman's correlation test.

These results – suggesting that progesterone may influence fibroid size – are supported by *in vivo* studies. If medroxyprogesterone acetate is given in combination with the GnRH agonist Zoladex®, then fibroid shrinkage fails to occur despite pituitary suppression[23]. However, if fibroid shrinkage is achieved using Zoladex® alone there is no increase in size if medroxyprogesterone acetate is then administered with the agonist. These results argue against an inhibitory effect of progesterone on fibroid growth and warrant further investigation.

THE ROLE OF GROWTH FACTORS

Although oestrogen action is important for fibroid growth, there is increasing evidence to suggest that the mitogenic effects of oestrogen may be mediated by local production of growth factors. The factors which have been most extensively studied in this context are epidermal growth factor (EGF), insulin-like growth factor (IGF) and transforming growth factor-β (TGF-β). Evidence for the hypothesis that oestrogen stimulates cell proliferation indirectly came initially from cell lines derived from oestrogen-responsive tumours or cell populations. An oestrogen-inducible rat uterine protein was reported to stimulate the proliferation of mammary, pituitary and kidney tumour cells[24]. Polypeptides related to EGF and IGF-I were detected in the serum-free medium of cultures of human breast cancer cells and treatment of MCF–7 breast cancer cells with 17β-oestradiol produced a fivefold increase of EGF-like activity in the medium[25]. The proliferation of mouse epithelial cells is enhanced by EGF, but not by other known growth factors, and the cells also contain high-affinity binding sites for EGF[26]. Human myometrium and fibroids contain high-affinity binding sites for EGF[27]. Although binding does not appear to vary during the menstrual cycle, the administration of Zoladex® induces a significant reduction in concentration[20] and the administration of oestradiol has the reverse effect[28]. Oestrogen has been shown to increase the relative rate of synthesis and accumulation of a protein (probably EGF) in the mouse uterus[29]. It appears to affect the rate of synthesis of the growth factor as well as affect the binding of the EGF to its receptor. Hybridization experiments have revealed the presence of a pre-pro-epidermal growth factor mRNA in the uterus, the concentration of which is influenced by oestrogen[30]. Pre-pro-EGF is the precursor of EGF and, possibly, oestradiol may stimulate the maturation process as well as the synthesis. The mRNA is present in very small concentrations and a specially modified polymerase-chain reaction is required to amplify it enough for identification and measurement. Oestradiol increases uterine EGF receptor mRNA levels *in vivo*[31]. This increase in the steady-state level of mRNA is likely to be the basis, at least in part, for the previously observed oestrogen-mediated increase in functional EGF receptor levels mentioned above. A very exciting study has been recently reported in which EGF was administered to oophorectomized mice[32]. Growth and differentiation of the female genital tract was achieved in the absence of oestrogen and even occurred in animals hypophysectomized and adrenalectomized as well[32]. This strongly suggests that EGF has an effect in mediating the stimulatory effects of oestrogen on the uterus.

There is also accumulating evidence that the insulin-like growth factors may have a role in the stimulation of fibroid growth. The regression of uterine and fibroid growth that is associated with the chronic administration of GnRH agonists is in turn associated with a significant reduction in circulating growth hormone and IGF-I[33]. However, this study failed to demonstrate any changes in IGF-II. It is possible that the secretion of IGF by fibroids and myometrium may exert an autocrine effect, since explant cultures of these tissues from women treated with GnRH agonist secrete significantly less IGF-I and IGF-II than tissues obtained from placebo treated controls[34]. Membranes from fibroids bind more IGF-I than myometrium[35] which suggests that locally produced factors may act on cells very near the site of production, as has been suggested with EGF above. It may also help explain why fibroids vary so much in size and growth potential. Insulin-like growth factor I mRNA is increased eight-fold by the administration of oestradiol[36]. This may explain the decrease in secretion with GnRH agonists, since it induces hypo-oestrogenism. Alternatively, growth hormone may be important, since it is considered to be a primary regulator of IGF-I secretion[37] as discussed in detail elsewhere. Follicle stimulating hormone stimulates insulin-like growth factor II mRNA production in human granulosa cells[38] and, therefore, the decreased secretion from myometrial explants may be related to the GnRH agonist effects on hormones other than oestradiol. Another possibility is that GnRH agonists cause an increase in cell death, because explants from agonist-treated women show decreased viability, compared with normal controls[34]. The uterus is an abundant source of both IGF-I and IGF-II[39] and the mRNA is present in leiomyomata.

Another interesting feature of fibroids is that they rarely become malignant. It is possible that this may be due to the presence of inhibitory growth factors such as TGF-β. I am not aware of any studies which have identified this factor in the human uterus, but tamoxifen increases its production from human breast cancer specimens[40]. Growth factors may alter the production of extracellular matrix, the structure of which may influence the invasive properties of a tumour, and this may provide one explanation, although it will be many years before the full answer is known.

SUMMARY

There is little doubt that oestrogen regulates the growth of uterine leiomyomata although the precise mode of action is unclear. The study of this mechanism is of considerable interest since it gives insight into hormonally controlled growth mechanisms, as well as the changes produced at an intracellular level by the steroid hormones.

REFERENCES

1. Jordan, V.C., Tate, A.C., Lyman, S.D., Gosden, B., Wolf, M.F., Bain, R.R. and Welshons, W.V. (1985). Rat uterine growth and induction of progesterone receptor without estrogen receptor translocation. *Endocrinology*, **116**, 1845–57
2. Green, S. and Chambon, P. (1991). The oestrogen receptor: from perception to mechanism. In Parker, M.G. (ed.) *Nuclear Hormone Receptors*, pp.15–38. (London: Academic Press)
3. Filicori, M., Hall, D.A., Loughlin, J.S., Rivier, J., Vale, W. and Crowley, W.F. (1983). A conservative approach to the management of uterine leiomyomata: pituitary desensitization by a luteinizing hormone-releasing

hormone analog. *Am. J. Obstet. Gynecol.*, **147**, 726–7

4. West, C.P., Lumsden, M.A., Lawson, S., Williamson, J. and Baird, D.T. (1987). Shrinkage of uterine fibroids during therapy with Zoladex (ICI 118630): a luteinizing hormone releasing hormone agonist administered as a monthly subcutaneous depot. *Fertil. Steril.*, **48**, 45–51
5. Farber, M., Conrad, S., Heinrichs, W. and Hermann, W. (1972). Estradiol binding by fibroid tumours and normal myometrium. *Obstet. Gynecol.*, **40**, 479–86
6. Puukka, M.J., Kontula, K.K., Kauppila, A.J., Janne, O.A. and Vikho, R.K. (1976). Estrogen receptor in human myoma tissue. *Mol. Cell. Endocrinol.*, **6**, 35–44
7. Wilson, E.A., Yang, F. and Rees, E.D. (1980). Estradiol and progesterone binding in uterine leiomyomata and in normal uterine tissues. *Obstet. Gynecol.*, **55**, 20–4
8. Lumsden, M.A., West, C.P., Hawkins, R.A., Bramley, T.A., Rumgay, L. and Baird, D.T. (1989). The binding of steroids to myometrium and leiomyomata (fibroids) in women treated with the gonadotrophin-releasing hormone agonist Zoladex (ICI 118630). *J. Endocrinol.*, **121**, 389–96
9. Gabb, R.G. and Stone, G.M. (1974). Uptake and metabolism of tritiated oestradiol and oestrone by human endometrium and myometrial tissue *in vitro*. *J. Endocrinol.*, **62**, 109–23
10. Tamaya, T., Motoyama, T., Ohnono, Y., Ide, N., Tsurusaki, T. and Okada, H. (1979). Estradiol-17β, progesterone and 5-dihydrotestosterone receptors of human myometrium and myoma in the human subject. *J. Steroid Biochem.*, **10**, 615–22
11. Bayard, F., Damilano, S., Robel, P. and Baulieu, E.E. (1978). Cytoplasmic and nuclear estradiol and progesterone receptors in human endometrium. *J. Clin. Endocrinol. Metab.*, **46**, 635–48
12. van der Walt, L., Sanfilippo, J.S., Siegel, J.E. and Wittliff, J.A. (1986). Estrogen and progestin receptors in human uterus: reference ranges of clinical conditions. *Clin. Physiol. Biochem.*, **4**, 217–28
13. Spellacy, W.N., LeMaire, W.J., Buhi, W.C., Birk, S.A. and Bradley, B.A. (1972). Plasma growth hormone and estradiol levels in women with uterine myomas. *Obstet. Gynecol.*, **40**, 829
14. Wiznitzer, A., Marbach, M., Hazum, E., Insler, V., Sharoni, Y. and Levy, T. (1988). Gonadotrophin-releasing hormone specific binding in uterine leiomyomata. *Biochem. Biophys. Res. Comm.*, **152**, 1326
15. Hawkins, R.A., Roberts, M.M. and Forrest, A.P. (1980). Oestrogen receptors and breast cancer: current status. *Br. J. Surg.*, **67**, 153–69
16. Goussard, J., Lechevrel, C., Martin, P.M. and Roussel, G. (1986). Comparison of monoclonal antibody and tritiated ligands for estrogen

receptor assays in 214 breast cancer cytosols. *Cancer Res.* (Suppl.) **46**, 4282–7s

17. Jordan, V.C., Jacobson, H.I. and Keenan, E.J. (1986). Determination of oestrogen receptor in breast cancer using monoclonal antibody technology: results of a multicenter study in the United States. *Cancer Res.* (Suppl.) **46**, 4237–40s
18. Leclerq, G., Bojar, H., Goussard, J., Nicholson, R.I., Richon, M.F., Piffanelli, A., Pousette, A., Thorpe, S. and Lonsdorfer, M. (1986). Abbott monoclonal enzyme immunoassay measurement of estrogen receptors in human breast cancer: a European multicenter study. *Cancer Res.* (Suppl.) **46**, 4233–6s
19. Sakai, F. and Saez, S. (1976). Existence of receptors bound to endogenous estradiol in breast cancers of premenopausal and postmenopausal women. *Steroids*, **27**, 99–110
20. Lumsden, M.A., West, C.P., Bramley, T., Rumgay, L. and Baird, D.T. (1988). The binding of epidermal growth factor to the human uterus and leiomyomata in women rendered hypoestrogenic by continuous administration of an LHRH agonist. *Br. J. Obstet. Gynaecol.*, **95**, 1299–1304
21. Levy, C., Robel, P., Gautray, J.P., DeBrux, J., Verma, U., Descomps, B. and Baulieu, E.E. (1980). Estradiol and progesterone receptors in human endometrium: normal and abnormal menstrual cycles and early pregnancy. *Am. J. Obstet. Gynecol.*, **136**, 646.
22. Schmidt-Gollwitzer, M., Gent, T., Schmidt-Gollwitzer, K., Pollow, B. and Pollow, K. (1978). In Brush, MG., King, R.J.B. and Taylor, R.W. (eds.) *Endometrial Cancer*, p.227. (London: Balliere Tindall)
23. West, C.P., Lumsden, M.A., Hillier, H., Sweeting, V. and Baird, D.T. (1992). Potential role for medroxy acetate as an adjunct to goserelin (Zoladex) in the medical management of uterine fibroids. *Hum. Reprod.*, in press
24. Sirbasku, D.A. (1978). Estrogen induction of growth factors specific for hormone-responsive mammary, pituitary and kidney tumor cells. *Proc. Natl. Acad. Sci. USA*, **75**, 3786
25. Dickson, R.B., Huff, K.K., Spencer, E.M. and Lippman, M.E. (1986). Induction of epidermal growth factor-related polypeptides by 17β-estradiol in MCF-7 human breast cancer cells. *Endocrinology*, **118**, 138–42
26. Tomooka, Y., Di Augustine, R.P. and McLachlan, J.A. (1986). Proliferation of mouse uterine epithelial cells *in vitro*. *Endocrinology*, **118**, 1011
27. Hofmann, D., Rao, C.L.V., Barrows, G.H., Schultz, G.S. and Sanfilippo, J.S. (1984). Binding sites for epidermal growth factor in human uterine tissues and leiomyomas. *J. Clin. Endocrinol. Metab.*, **58**, 880–4
28. Mikku, V.R. and Stancel, G.M. (1985). Regulation of epidermal growth

factor receptor by oestrogen. *J. Biol. Chem.*, **260**, 9820–4

29. Huet-Hudson, Y.M., Chakraborty, C., De, S.K., Suzuki, Y., Andrews, G.K. and Dey, S.K. (1990). Estrogen regulates the synthesis of epidermal growth factor in mouse uterine epithelial cells. *Mol. Endocrinol.*, **4**, 510–23
30. Di Augustine, R.P., Petrusz, P., Bell, G.I., Brown, C.F., Korach, K.S., McLachlan, J.A. and Teng, C.T. (1988). Influence of estrogens on mouse uterine epidermal growth factor precursor protein and messenger ribonucleic acid. *Endocrinology*, **122**, 2355–63
31. Lingham, R.B., Stancel, G.M. and Loose-Mitchell, D.S. (1988). Estrogen regulation of epidermal growth factor receptor messenger ribonucleic acid. *Mol. Endocrinol.*, **2**, 230–5
32. Nelson, K.G., Takahashi, T., Bossert, N.L., Walmer, D.K. and McLachlan, J.A. (1991). Epidermal growth factor replaces estrogen in the stimulation of female genital tract growth and differentiation. *Proc. Natl. Acad. Sci. USA*, **88**, 21–5
33. Friedman, A.J., Rein, M.S., Pandian, M.R. and Barbieri, R.L. (1990). Fasting serum growth hormone and insulin-like growth factor-I and -II concentrations in women with leiomyomata uteri treated with leuprolide acetate or placebo. *Fertil. Steril.*, **53**, 250–3
34. Rein, M.S., Friedman, A.J., Pandian, M.R. and Heffner, L.J. (1990). The secretion of insulin-like growth factors I and II by explant cultures of fibroids and myometrium from women treated with a gonadotropin-releasing hormone agonist. *Obstet. Gynecol.*, **76**, 388–94
35. Tommola, P., Pekonen, F. and Rutanen, E.M. (1989). Binding of epidermal growth factor I in human myometrium and leiomyomata. *Obstet. Gynecol.*, **74**, 658–62
36. Norstedt, G., Levinovitz, A. and Eriksson, H. (1989). Regulation of uterine insulin-like growth factor I mRNA and insulin-like growth factor II mRNA by estrogen in the rat. *Acta Endocrinol. (Copenh.)*, **120**, 466–72
37. Matthews, L.S., Norstedt, G. and Palmer, R.D. (1986). Regulation of insulin-like growth factor 1 gene expression by growth hormone. *Proc. Natl. Acad. Sci. USA*, **83**, 9343–7
38. Voutilainen, R. and Miller, W.L. (1987). Coordinate tropic hormone regulation of mRNAs for insulin-like growth factor II and the cholesterol side-chain-cleavage enzyme, P450ssc in human steroidogenic tissues. *Proc. Natl. Acad. Sci. USA*, **84**, 1590–4
39. Murphy, L.J., Bell, G.I. and Friesen, H.J. (1987). Tissue distribution of insulin-like growth factor I and II messenger ribonucleic acid in the adult rat. *Endocrinology*, **120**, 1279–82
40. Wang, J.L. and Hsu, Y.M. (1986). Negative regulators of cell growth. *TIBS*, **2**, 24–6

3

Uterine fibroids: histological features

J. Crow

INTRODUCTION

Studies of the distribution of glucose-6-phosphate dehydrogenase isoenzymes in uterine fibroids of mosaic individuals[1] have shown that each lesion contains only one enzyme type. This has been taken to indicate that they are monoclonal proliferations and are therefore considered to be true benign neoplasms of myometrial smooth muscle and should correctly be termed leiomyomas. They are the commonest tumours seen in most diagnostic histopathology departments. They are frequently multiple and vary in size from less than 1 cm to very large masses which are often of extremely hard consistency. They are generally well circumscribed but not encapsulated and often have a plane of cleavage around the periphery which may be visible both macroscopically and microscopically. They have a typically white, whorled cut surface.

GENERAL HISTOLOGICAL FEATURES

Microscopically, leiomyomas are composed of interlacing bundles of elongated smooth muscle fibres with cigar-shaped nuclei and eosinophilic cytoplasm, surrounded by variable amounts of collagenous fibrous tissue (Figure 1). Within this fibrous tissue are blood vessels of various sizes and also variable numbers of mast cells which may be demonstrated by special staining techniques. Visible degenerative changes which may be seen

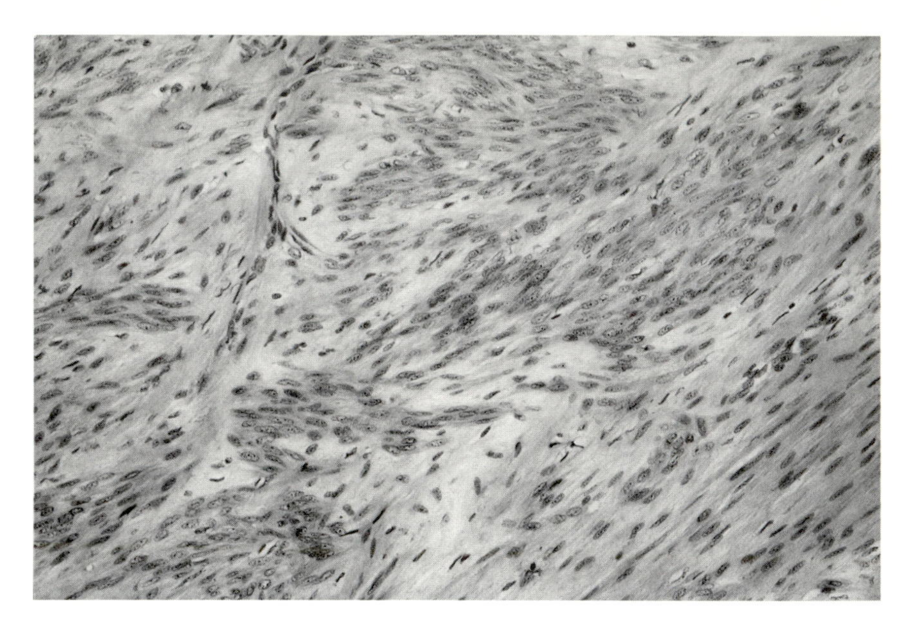

Figure 1 Leiomyoma from untreated case showing interlacing bundles of smooth muscle fibres surrounded by fibrous tissue (H&E; x126)

commonly include hyalinization of the collagenous component, myxoid and cystic changes, and calcification. These are probably of little clinical significance but a more dramatic change is haemorrhagic infarction, which may occur particularly during pregnancy.

Histologically, the most important distinction to make is the difference from the equivalent malignant tumour, the leiomyosarcoma. This tumour is relatively rare and not usually difficult to recognize with its high cellularity, nuclear pleomorphism, high mitotic rate with abnormal mitoses, areas of necrosis and infiltrating margins. However, there are some smooth muscle tissue tumours with pleomorphism which are not malignant and some cases with intermediate numbers of mitoses whose malignant potential is unpredictable (Table 1)[2,3].

ULTRASTRUCTURAL FEATURES

Under the electron microscope the smooth muscle cells of the tumours are surrounded by a greater amount of collagen than those of normal

Table 1 Features of uterine smooth muscle tumours

Mitotic figures (per 10 high-power fields)	*Increased cellularity*	*Atypia*	*Diagnosis*
0–4	–	–	Usual leiomyoma
0–4	+	–	Cellular leiomyoma
0–4	+	+	Symplastic leiomyoma
5–9	+	–	Uncertain malignant potential
5–9	+	+	Leiomyosarcoma
>10	+	– or +	Leiomyosarcoma

myometrium[4] but otherwise look very similar. The characteristic features are an elongated nucleus with indented margins and an open chromatin pattern, and extensive cytoplasm containing the longitudinally orientated microfilaments with randomly distributed dense bodies that make up the contractile apparatus of the cell (Figure 2). Only a few other organelles are usually visible. At the cell membrane there are numerous dense plaques for the insertion of the microfilaments[5] and these are interspersed with collections of pinocytotic vesicles which are concerned with the uptake of fluid from the extracellular space. Immediately outside the cell membrane is a layer of external lamina and surrounding the cells are the characteristic banded fibres of collagen.

MAST CELLS

Mast cells are very widely distributed in the connective tissue of many organs but their presence in leiomyomas is of interest as they may sometimes be very numerous and their granules contain physiologically active substances including histamine and heparin. In view of the common clinical presentation with menorrhagia, which is of uncertain pathogenesis[6], an assessment of the numbers of mast cells in leiomyomas has been carried out as part of a larger study of the distribution of these cells in the female genital tract[7].

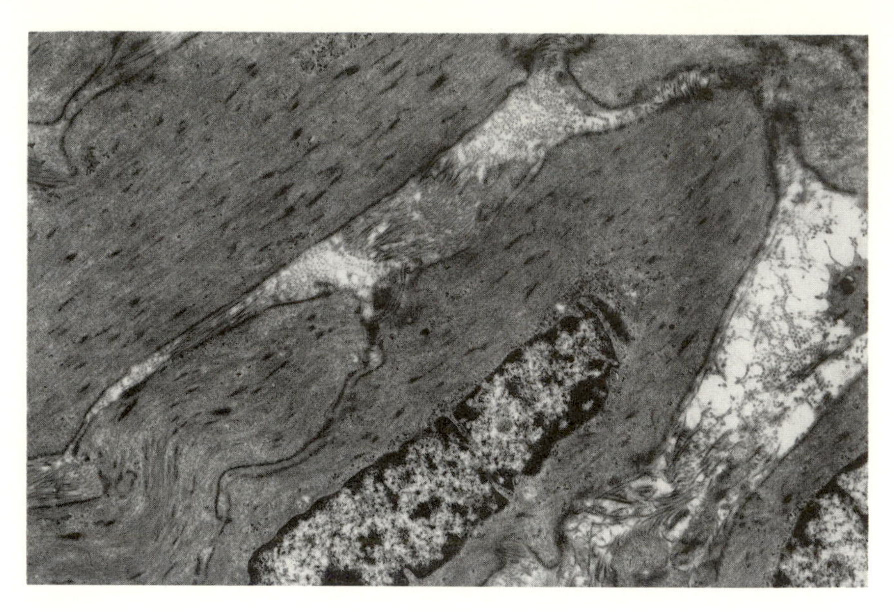

Figure 2 Ultrastructure of untreated leiomyoma showing cells containing cytoplasmic microfilaments with focal densities and surface plaques surrounded by collagen fibres (x5400)

The mean counts were found generally to be lower in leiomyomas (range 0–43 mast cells/mm^2) than in the adjacent myometrium (range 8–128 mast cells/mm^2). No relationship was found between the numbers of mast cells in leiomyomas and the age of the patient, the menopause, menorrhagia as a presenting symptom, the site of the tumour, the size of the tumour or the amount of collagen present within the lesion. There was also no significant difference in counts in the myometrial samples between cases with and without leiomyomas. There was no difference in the mast cell counts between samples taken from the centre or the periphery of the larger lesions but there was some relationship to overall cellularity with high counts being found in some cellular leiomyomas and a particularly high count of 312 mast cells/mm^2 in a densely cellular lesion from a patient who had been treated by Zoladex® (Figure 3).

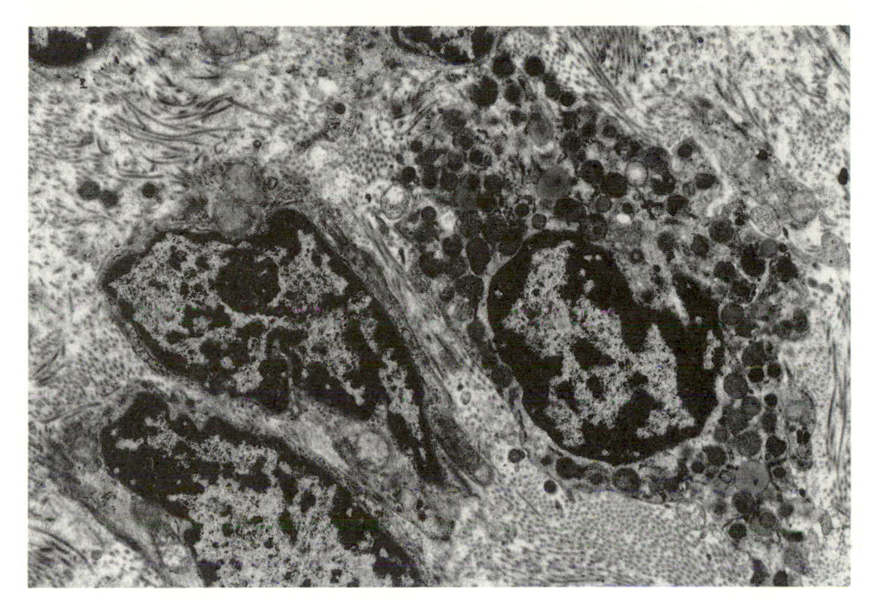

Figure 3 Mast cell with cytoplasmic granules adjacent to small tumour cells with little evidence of myofibrillar differentiation; from case *Qu* which showed marked cellular crowding, including large numbers of mast cells (x6340)

EFFECTS OF TREATMENT BY GnRH ANALOGUE

A detailed histological and ultrastructural study has been made of leiomyomas from patients treated with Zoladex® together with untreated control cases in order to document the morphological changes in the tumours. The findings have been correlated with the ultrasound measurements of uterine shrinkage and attempts have been made to identify the causes of variation in response between different patients.

Patients and methods

Nine patients were treated with Zoladex® (goserelin, ICI 118630) four doses of 3.6 mg subcutaneously monthly, starting in the early follicular phase of the cycle. Both these patients and eight untreated controls had uterine volume determinations made from ultrasound measurements before and after the treatment period. The patients then underwent either myomectomy or hysterectomy and samples of the leiomyomas were taken for both light and electron microscopic examination.

Table 2 Variables measured in patients with uterine leiomyomas treated by Zoladex®

Case	*Volume loss* (cm³)	*Volume shrinkage* (%)	*Age* (years)	*Original size* (cm³)	*Nuclear area* (mm² x 10³)	*Collagen area* (mm² x 10³)	*Vessel area* (mm² x 10³)
Ab	183.7	48.4	38	379.9	20.9	145.2	—
Ad	49.8	13.3	38	373.6	—	267.7	—
Br	86.4	20.5	40	421.1	18.8	270.1	4.2
Do	49.7	40.3	36	123.2	83.6	13.7	11.8
Du	230.8	36.2	49	637.4	26.4	187.0	9.5
Pa	299.0	31.8	43	938.5	29.6	229.9	5.5
Ph	287.5	33.7	33	852.9	22.5	303.7	5.1
Ro	86.7	51.3	48	169.0	17.0	263.5	3.2
Qu	198.7	18.6	36	1069.4	78.9	123.7	6.8

As well as routine haematoxylin and eosin staining, Van Gieson stain was used in the assessment of the collagen content whilst haematoxylin with no counterstain was used for the assessment of nuclear crowding and an immunohistological technique using *QBend*© antibody was used to stain vascular endothelium for the assessment of vascularity. Videomorphometry was carried out using the Chromatic Colour Image Analysis System[8]. The results were analysed using the Spearman rank–order correlation coefficient. Further morphological observations were made on hysterectomy specimens from other similarly treated cases, including two treated by a 3-month depot preparation of Zoladex®.

RESULTS

Histological features

Despite the fact that all the treated cases had shown some degree of uterine shrinkage over the treatment period (Table 2), the histological appearances were very variable. Two cases (*Do* and *Qu*) showed extreme crowding of nuclei which produced a densely cellular appearance (Figure 4) but with no evidence of mitotic activity. On the other hand, six of the patients showed no cellular crowding and there was no significant difference between the nuclear area measurements of these cases and the untreated controls.

In the ninth treated case (*Ad*), nuclear crowding of the tumour cells could not be measured objectively because there were significant numbers of inflammatory cells (mainly lymphocytes) within the lesion. This was not a feature found in any of the control cases although after a specific search two of the other treated cases (*Ab* and *Qu*) were found to have a few such cells. Further emphasis is placed on this finding with the discovery that both the depot-treated cases also showed lymphoid cell infiltration and one of the other leiomyomas in the hysterectomy of patient *Ab* showed a very marked infiltrate with formation of lymphoid follicles (Figure 5). The cells in this case were identified as B lymphocytes (L26 positive) and plasma cells of both the κ and λ light chain type.

The results of the morphometric measurements are shown in Table 2 in relation to the original size of the uterus, the absolute volume decrease of the uterus over the treatment period, the degree of shrinkage as a percentage of the original size and the age of the patient at the time of surgery.

Statistical analysis of these various factors has shown only one significant positive correlation with uterine shrinkage. The decrease in uterine volume after treatment shows a correlation ($p < 0.01$) with the original size of the uterus; in other words, the larger the uterus was originally, the greater the decrease in volume obtained by Zoladex® treatment. None of the histologically measured variables showed a significant correlation with either the absolute volume loss or the degree of shrinkage, although there was a negative correlation ($p < 0.05$) between the nuclear crowding and the area of collagen in the histological sections.

Examination of hysterectomy specimens from treated cases has revealed no difference in the apparent size of the perimyomatous plane of cleavage compared with untreated cases.

Electron microscopy

The ultrastructural features were also quite variable from case to case. The most severe changes were seen in case *Do* which showed small cells with minimal residual myofibrillar structures and considerable degenerative changes. In places, the damaged cytoplasmic organelles were seen in direct

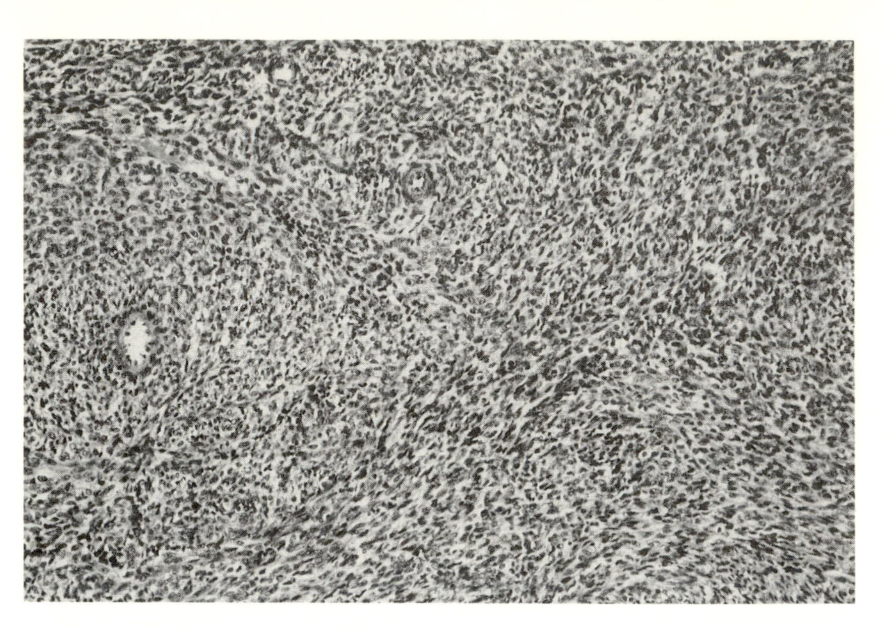

Figure 4 One of the two leiomyomas (case *Do*) which showed marked crowding of cells after GnRH analogue treatment (H&E; ×126)

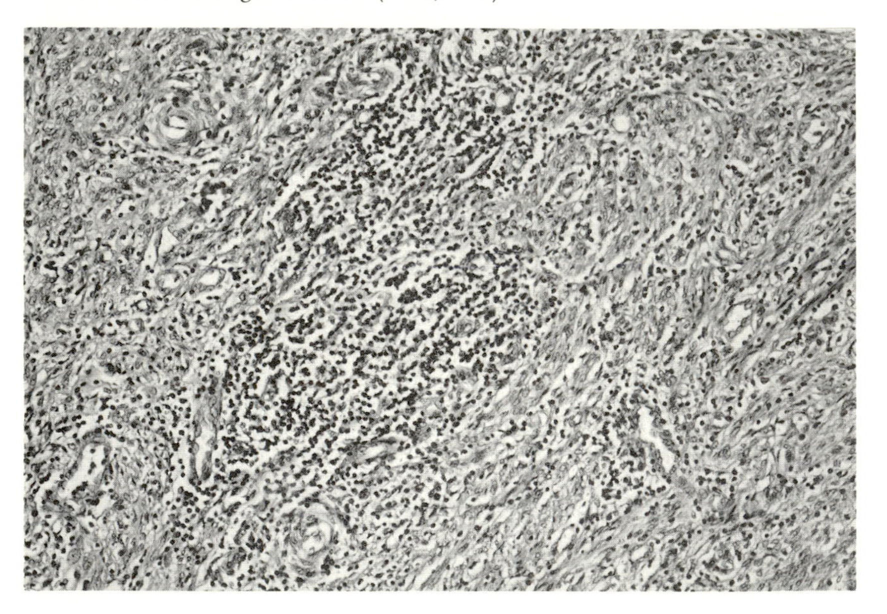

Figure 5 Leiomyoma from a hysterectomy specimen (case *Ab*) which showed marked lymphoid cell infiltration following GnRH analogue treatment (H&E; ×126)

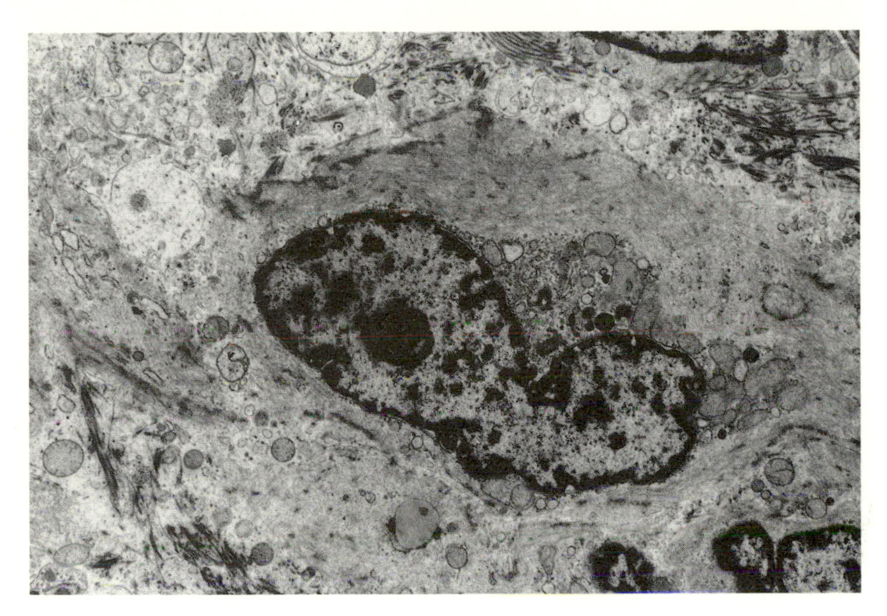

Figure 6 Ultrastructure of leiomyoma from case *Do* showing a small cell with inconspicuous, rather disordered microfilaments and cell disruption with cytoplasmic organelles immediately adjacent to collagen fibres (x5540)

continuity with collagen fibres indicating that cell surface membranes had been disrupted (Figure 6).

Case *Qu* also showed very small cells with only small areas of rather disorganized myofibrillar differentiation and relatively greater numbers of other cytoplasmic organelles. A few cytoplasmic vacuoles were present but in this case the cell membranes appeared intact. The marked cellular crowding in this lesion was also reflected in the very large numbers of mast cells visible at both the light and electron microscopic level (Figure 3).

In several cases the leiomyoma cells generally showed no particularly abnormal ultrastructural features and had well preserved myofibrillar apparatus, but variable numbers of cells contained partially membrane-bound compound lysosomal structures which were presumed to have been formed from degenerated intracellular organelles. This feature was most marked in case *Ro* who started with a fairly small uterus and showed the highest percentage shrinkage after treatment (Figure 7). Case *Ad*, which showed lymphocyte infiltration in the leiomyoma, did not exhibit degenerative changes in the tumour cells.

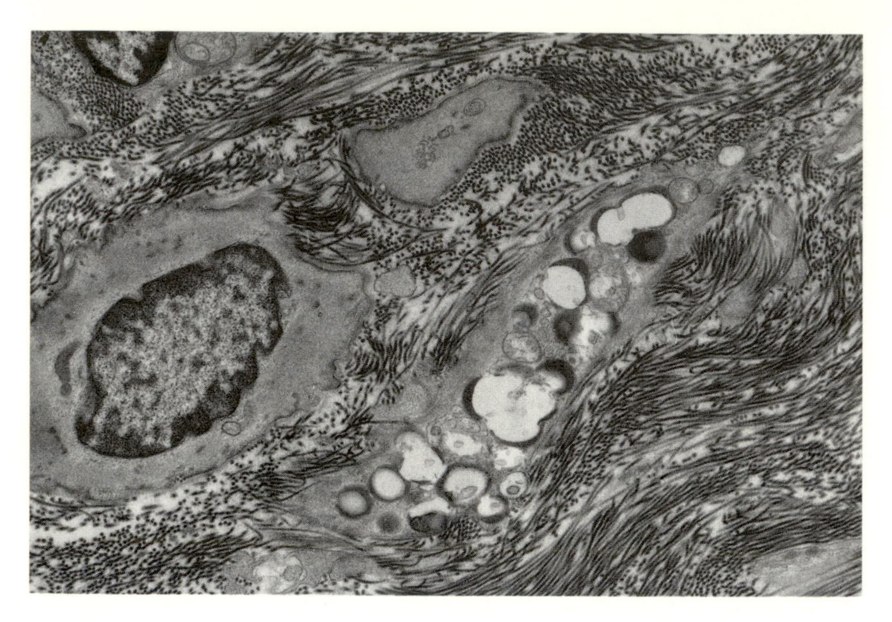

Figure 7 Prominent compound lysosomal bodies in a tumour cell from case *Ro* (x7920)

Ultrastructural examination was carried out on both leiomyoma and myometrium from one of the cases treated by depot preparation. The leiomyoma showed crowded small cells with disorganized myofilaments, vacuolation and lysosomal bodies, whereas in the myometrium the cells were not significantly abnormal.

DISCUSSION

In summary, the morphological changes which have been identified in leiomyomas after GnRH analogue therapy are: a variable degree of shrinkage and crowding of leiomyoma cells with loss of ultrastructural evidence of smooth muscle differentiation, together with a variable degree of cytoplasmic damage and formation of lysosomal residual bodies. In addition, some cases showed an infiltrate of chronic inflammatory cells (mainly lymphocytes). However, some cases showed very little change from untreated leiomyomas.

The most remarkable feature of these results is the pronounced degree of variation in appearance between different cases, at both the light and electron microscopical level. No good reason has emerged to explain this. One plausible suggestion – that the greater the amount of collagen within a tumour the less it is able to shrink – appears to be true for the areas sampled histologically, but does not correlate with the overall uterine shrinkage measurements; neither does the vascularity (as measured histologically) appear to affect the outcome. Even more surprising is the fact that of the two cases which appeared very shrunken histologically, one was from the smallest uterus (patient *Do*) which showed a high percentage shrinkage, whereas the other (patient *Qu*) was from the largest uterus which showed only a modest degree of shrinkage. Thus, there is not even a good correlation between the histological evidence of shrinkage and the ultrasonographic measurements. A possible explanation for this could be the quite marked variation in appearance, particularly after treatment, between different tumours in one uterus and even between different areas of a single lesion (Figure 8). Consequently, the histological sample of one small area of one lesion may not correlate at all well with the overall effects on the whole uterus. This still leaves the problem of why some lesions or parts of lesions respond more than others. A variable collagen content may be part of the reason but it could also involve the growth phase of the tumour and/or the variable concentrations of oestrogen receptors[9]. Without a pretreatment sample it would be difficult to test these hypotheses histologically.

The presence of a lymphoid cell infiltrate in some cases is of interest. It does not appear to correlate with the degree of cell damage present and, indeed, damaged cells would be expected to elicit a neutrophil polymorphonuclear acute inflammatory type of reaction rather than a lymphocytic response, the implication of which is an immunological reaction. Possibly, the changes at the cell surface involve alteration to surface antigens, thereby eliciting such an immune response. In any case, the effect may be to mitigate any shrinkage effects of the therapy because of the increased size caused by the infiltrating inflammatory cell population.

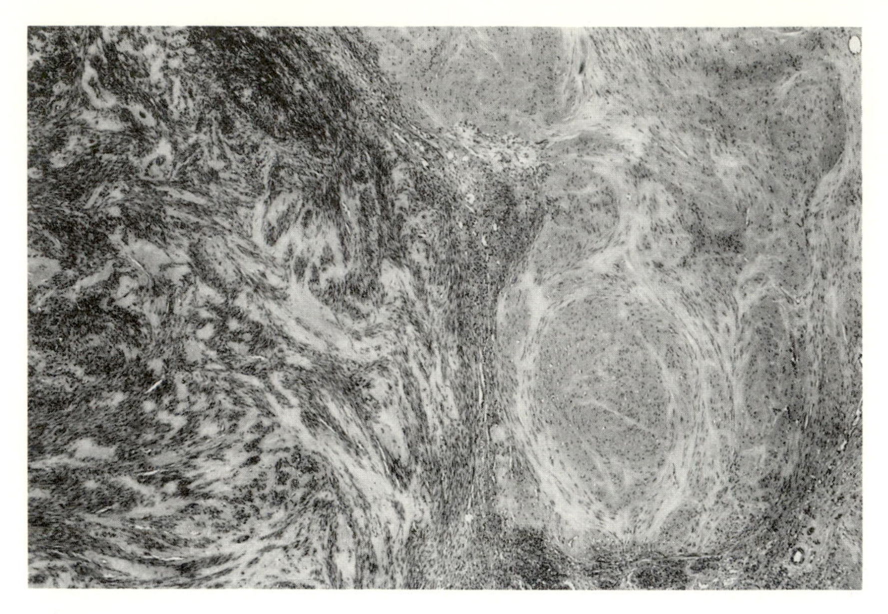

Figure 8 Leiomyoma from treated case showing adjacent areas of very different cellularity (H&E; x32)

CONCLUSIONS

Uterine leiomyomas are extremely common benign tumours providing plentiful material for histological study. Although apparently of boring uniformity, their structure varies considerably between areas and hence measurements of histological features are fraught with sampling problems. A study of their content of mast cells has revealed that their variable number may be partly a reflection of their overall cellularity, and does not provide evidence to suggest that they are involved in the pathogenesis of associated menorrhagia. A study of the effects of GnRH analogue treatment has shown highly variable degrees of cell shrinkage and cytoplasmic damage, together with a lymphoid cell infiltrate in some cases.

REFERENCES

1. Townsend, D.E., Sparkes, R.S., Baluda, M.C. and McClelland, G. (1970). Unicellular histogenesis of uterine leiomyomas as determined by electrophoresis of glucose-6-phosphate dehydrogenase. *Am. J. Obstet. Gynecol.*, **107**, 1168–73
2. Norris, H.J. and Zaloudek, C.J. (1982). Mesenchymal tumours of the uterus. In Blaustein, A. (ed.) *Pathology of the Female Genital Tract*, pp.352–92. (New York: Springer-Verlag)
3. Kempson, R.L. and Hendrickson, M.R. (1988). Pure mesenchymal neoplasms of the uterine corpus. *Sem. Diagn. Pathol.*, **5**, 172–98
4. Ferenczy, A. and Richart, R.C. (1971). A comparative ultrastructural study of leiomyosarcoma, cellular leiomyoma and leiomyoma of the uterus. *Cancer*, **28**, 1004–18
5. Hopkins, C.R. (1978). Microfilaments and muscle contraction: smooth muscle. In Hopkins, C.R. *Structure and Function of Cells*, pp.216–21. (London: W.B. Saunders)
6. Buttram, V.C. and Reiter, R.C. (1981). Uterine leiomyomata: aetiology, symptomatology and management. *Fertil. Steril.*, **36**, 433–45
7. Crow, J., Wilkins, M., Howe, S., More, L. and Helliwell, P. (1991). Mast cells in the female genital tract. *Int. J. Gynecol. Pathol.*, **10** 230–7
8. Jarvis, L.R. (1986). A microcomputer system for video analysis and diagnostic microdensitometry. *Anal. Quant. Cytol. Histol.*, **8**, 201–9
9. Rein, M.S., Friedmann, A.J., Stuart, J.M. and MacLaughlin, D.T. (1990). Fibroid and myometrial steroid receptors in women treated with gonadotrophin-releasing hormone agonist leuprolide acetate. *Fertil. Steril.*, **53**, 1018–23

4

Uterine fibroids: clinical presentation and diagnostic techniques

C.P. West

CLINICAL PRESENTATION

Uterine fibroids are estimated to affect at least 20% of women of reproductive age, with well recognized racial differences influencing their prevalence. It seems likely that as many as 50% of affected women are asymptomatic[1] although many otherwise asymptomatic fibroids may be discovered during routine pelvic or antenatal examination. In this situation, presentation is affected by the age and reproductive status of the individual as well as by the site of origin of the fibroids. For example, smallish fibroids associated with no menstrual upset are more likely to be detected in a woman attending for the investigation of infertility or for routine antenatal care than in a woman who has completed childbearing. However, prevalence rises with increasing age. The site of fibroids, rather than their size, affects presentation and very large subserous tumours may be asymptomatic, in contrast to the marked menstrual upset associated with relatively small submucous fibroids. A detailed review of the clinical presentation of uterine fibroids has been published by Buttram and Reiter[1] and the subject is covered in standard gynaecological textbooks, so that references in this text will be confined to those required to qualify specific points.

COMPLICATIONS

It could be argued that all symptomatic presentations represent complications arising from fibroids developing in various sites, rather than as an inevitable consequence of their presence. The commonest symptomatic presentation is with menorrhagia, reported by around 30% of women with fibroids, although the mechanism of the abnormal blood loss is unclear (see the review by West and Lumsden[2]). Fibroids are commonly associated with childlessness and low parity (see the review by Buttram and Reiter[1]) although their actual contribution to subfertility is controversial.

Pregnancy-related fibroids

Uterine fibroids may present with symptoms for the first time during pregnancy or asymptomatic fibroids may be detected clinically or by ultrasonography. The complications of spontaneous abortion, premature labour, malpresentation and obstructed labour have been well described (Table 1). In a large population study based on routine antenatal ultrasound examination, it was estimated that around 2% of pregnancies occur in women with fibroids[3]. However, only 10% of the women in the latter series were admitted with complications related to their fibroids. The majority of these admissions were with pain attributable to red degeneration, associated with ultrasound appearances of heterogeneous echo patterns and cystic spaces, and characteristically occurring in the mid-trimester of pregnancy. Of the 28 women admitted with complications, the same authors reported six (21%) with spontaneous premature rupture of membranes, leading to mid-trimester pregnancy loss in two and early delivery in the other four. In a similar review of pregnancy complications, Muram and colleagues[4] reported an early spontaneous abortion rate which was no higher than that of the normal obstetric population but confirmed a higher prevalence of premature membrane rupture. They found that the latter complication, together with bleeding and pregnancy loss, was associated with a close proximity between placental site and fibroids and that placental location, rather than fibroid size, was the main predictor of pregnancy outcome. In theory, the presence of uterine fibroids might be implicated as a cause of placental insufficiency and intrauterine foetal growth retardation but this does not

Table 1 Pregnancy complications

Phase	*Complication*
Early	?Pregnancy loss
Mid-trimester	Spontaneous rupture of membranes Pregnancy loss Red degeneration
Late	Spontaneous rupture of membranes Preterm labour Malpresentation Obstructed labour Postpartum haemorrhage

appear to be supported in the literature. Contrary to established belief, serial ultrasound monitoring of fibroid size in pregnancy[5] shows that the majority of fibroids do not enlarge during pregnancy.

Pressure symptoms

Less common presentations are with complications related to the varied sites of origin and to the position of the fibroids (Table 2). Site of origin also influences the size which a fibroid can attain before it gives rise to clinical problems, including effects of pressure or impingement on surrounding structures. Bowel complications have rarely been reported but urinary symptoms include frequency of micturition related to pressure from anterior fibroids, retention of urine where a fibroid arises from the cervix or ureteric obstruction with cervical or large broad ligament fibroids. Pedunculated subserous fibroids may present as an acute abdomen if torsion or haemorrhage occurs. Rarely, detachment (resulting in a so-called 'parasitic' fibroid) has led to diagnostic confusion, and may be associated with ascites. Submucous fibroids seldom achieve a large size but may become ulcerated and infected, particularly if prolapsed. A large submucous fibroid may often present with painful expulsion through the cervix, mimicking labour and, in rare cases, this may lead to uterine inversion.

Table 2 Complications relating to site of origin

Site	*Complication*
Any	Pressure/impingement (related to size)
Cervical	Urinary retention Ureteric obstruction
Subserous	Broad ligament Torsion Haemorrhage Parasitic fibroids
Submucous	Ulceration/infection Prolapse/expulsion

Haematological complications

These most commonly take the form of iron deficiency anaemia, secondary to menorrhagia and the anaemia is not infrequently the symptom which draws attention to the presence of fibroids in women with a low threshold for complaint. Paradoxically, fibroids may be associated with polycythaemia, reportedly due to the inappropriate secretion of erythropoietin by fibroid tissue[6].

Degenerative changes

Such changes are thought to be an inevitable occurrence in fibroids as they enlarge, although only the complication of red degeneration in pregnancy, described above, is associated with a well-described symptomatic presentation. In a review of 298 cases treated surgically, no correlation was found between presenting symptoms and histological evidence of degenerative changes[7]. Vollenhoven and colleagues[8] reported two cases of acute pain which necessitated hospitalization during GnRH analogue treatment. One of these was associated with prolapse of a large infarcted submucous fibroid polyp and we have experience of a similar case[2]. It is presumed that this complication is related to acute vascular necrosis, secondary to oestrogen deprivation. Calcification occurs commonly as a later consequence of circulatory impairment, such as in the case of subserous fibroids with narrow pedicles, and is a characteristic occurrence after the menopause when fibroids may present for the first time as incidental calcified masses on abdominal X-rays.

Malignant changes

Sarcomatous change is potentially lethal but thought to be extremely rare[1,9]. The authors of the latter studies estimate an incidence of no more than 0.1% in women with fibroids. Earlier higher figures were thought to be biased by the inclusion of cases of leiomyosarcoma which did not arise in pre-existing fibroids, and by the failure to take into consideration the high incidence of asymptomatic fibroids in most populations. This tumour is more common postmenopausally, presenting most frequently with painful uterine enlargement or bleeding; suspicion must always be alerted if there is documented spontaneous uterine enlargement or tenderness in a postmenopausal woman. In contrast to malignancy, another unusual complication of uterine fibroids is so-called intravenous leiomyomatosis, a benign spread of fibroid nodules into the pelvic veins, with occasional metastases in distant structures, such as the lung[10].

INVESTIGATIONS

Before the advent of current diagnostic techniques, diagnosis of uterine fibroids was largely clinical, necessitating early surgical intervention in a large proportion of cases because of the difficulty in distinguishing between uterine enlargement and the presence of ovarian neoplasia. Recent developments have not only aided diagnosis but have also led to the development of a wider range of therapeutic options, and have increased the scope for conservative management and medical therapy because of the facility for accurate monitoring.

Hysterosalpingography and laparoscopy

Hysterosalpingography is used to delineate the degree of uterine cavity distortion in women with known or suspected fibroids who desire pregnancy or have a history of pregnancy loss. It also gives useful information about tubal patency, particularly in cases where submucous fibroids are encroaching on the tubal cornu and, in some centres, it is used as a primary procedure in the investigation of subfertility. Many small, asymptomatic, intramural or subserous fibroids are detected for the first time during diagnostic laparoscopy, particularly when carried out for the investigation of subfertility or less commonly in women undergoing sterilization or other laparoscopic procedures. Diagnostic laparoscopy has a particularly useful role in the clarification of the nature of small pelvic masses. Laparoscopic techniques for the removal of small fibroids have been described, although the role of such intervention in the overall clinical management of women with fibroids is currently unclear.

Ultrasonography

Diagnostic ultrasonography is the most widely utilized procedure for the investigation and diagnosis of pelvic masses (Figure 1). There have been a number of published reports of studies which have evaluated the accuracy of abdominal ultrasound diagnosis, comparing ultrasound appearances with operative findings and definitive pathological diagnosis. In four large series[12–15], each reporting over 200 cases (1026 in total), the nature and site of a pelvic mass was predicted with accuracy in over 80% of cases and 227 out of 257 diagnoses of uterine fibroids (88%) were predicted correctly (Table 3). In most cases where the diagnosis of fibroids was uncertain or incorrect, this was attributable to the small size of the fibroids or the difficulty in distinguishing between pedunculated subserous or broad ligament fibroids and solid ovarian tumours. One uterine sarcoma was incorrectly diagnosed as a fibroid. Abdominal ultrasound may not detect small fibroids but the latter problem can now be overcome using a vaginal probe, which also improves visualization of the ovaries so that improved accuracy with current techniques can be anticipated. For routine diagnostic purposes, accurate measurement of the size of fibroids is not necessary but this is important where ultrasonographic monitoring

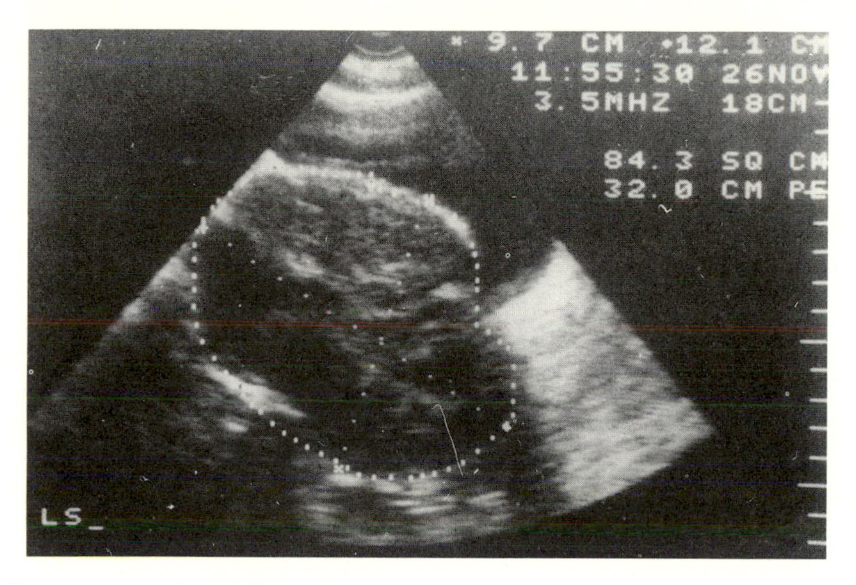

Figure 1 An enlarged fibroid uterus as demonstrated by ultrasound. (Courtesy of Prof. R.W. Shaw, from reference 11, with permission)

Table 3 Accuracy of abdominal ultrasound: 1026 pelvic masses

Number of fibroids	*Diagnosis correct*	*Authors*
52	45 (86%)	Cochrane and Thomas (1974)[12]
152	142 (93%)	Levi and Delval (1976)[13]
19	17 (89%)	Lawson and Albarelli (1977)[14]
34	23 (68%)	Walsh and colleagues (1977)[15]
257	227 (88%)	All studies

is used during conservative management or in assessing response to therapy – for example with GnRH analogues. The volume of the uterus or of individual fibroids can be calculated using the formula $\frac{4}{3}\pi r^3$. In a study of over 60 women, the volume of the surgically removed uterus was measured by water displacement and compared with the immediate preoperative measurement of total uterine volume obtained by ultrasonography, we found a highly significant correlation between the two methods[16].

Magnetic resonance imaging

Magnetic resonance imaging (MRI) is a newer technique which offers advantages over ultrasonography in terms of improved imaging quality and accuracy (Figure 2). In a study of 23 women undergoing hysterectomy, MRI scans performed 14 days before surgery identified correctly 58 out of 59 individual fibroids, the smallest with a diameter of 0.3 cm (Table 4)[17]. One large submucous fibroid was incorrectly diagnosed as an endometrial carcinoma. The same authors were able to study the correlation between signal intensity and the histological features of individual fibroids, and identified two main subgroups. Fibroids with a homogeneous low signal intensity were invariably small (< 6 cm diameter) and histologically were composed of smooth muscle with no degenerative changes. Those showing heterogeneous patterns were larger and, histologically, contained degenerative changes but the features were non-specific. These patterns were not found to predict degree of response to GnRH analogues[18]. Compared with ultrasonography, which has the advantage of a high acceptability to patients, low cost and wide availability, MRI is extremely costly and currently limited in its application. It is usually reserved for cases of diagnostic difficulty and as a research tool.

Hysteroscopy

Another technique which has gained considerable popularity by virtue of its therapeutic and diagnostic potential is direct endoscopic visualization by hysteroscopy. It is most often used for the investigation of menstrual dysfunction when small, otherwise unsuspected submucous fibroids may be identified, giving a higher yield of abnormalities compared with conventional curettage[19]. However, endometrial histology – whether obtained by conventional curettage or biopsy – must not be overlooked as an essential part of the investigation of any woman with abnormal (particularly irregular) bleeding, even where fibroids have been clearly

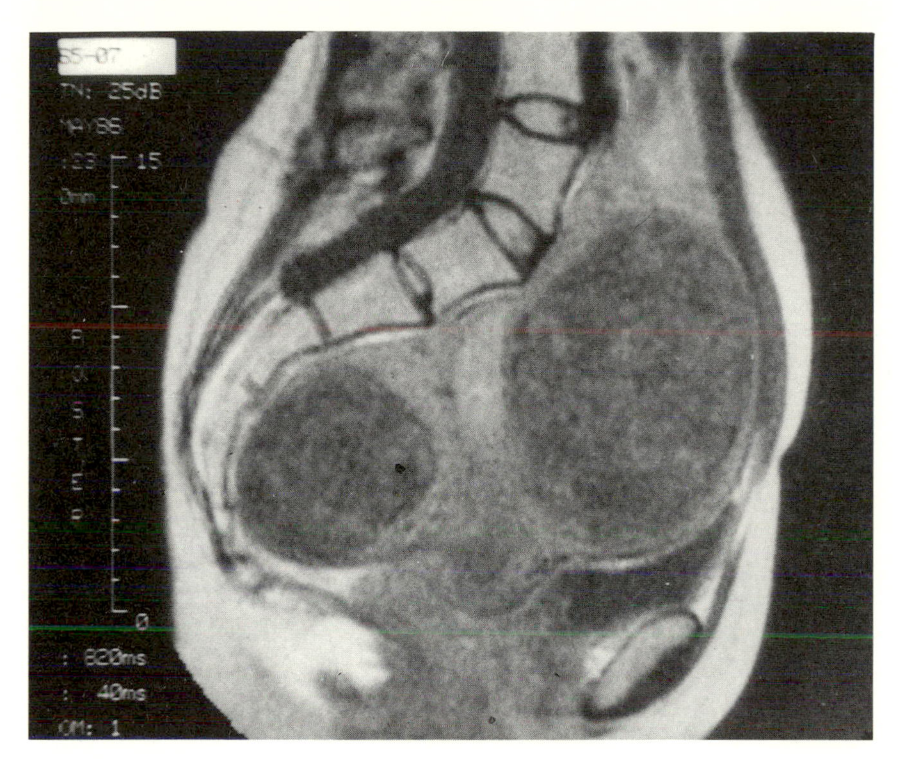

Figure 2 The increased clarity of definition of a fibroid uterus as visualized by magnetic resonance imaging (same patient as Figure 1). (Courtesy of Prof. R.W. Shaw, from reference 11, with permission)

Table 4 Magnetic resonance imaging in uterine fibroids. Data from a study of 23 women by Hricak and colleagues (1986)[17]

Site	*Present*	*Correct*
Subserosal	9	9
Broad ligament	1	1
Cervical	1	1
Intramural	37	37
Submucosal	11	10*
Total	59	58

*Misdiagnosed as endometrial carcinoma

identified because of the risk of coincidental endometrial pathology. Hysteroscopy is also useful in the investigation of subfertility and recurrent pregnancy loss and may be required to clarify the nature of small uterine filling defects identified by hysterosalpingography. The endoscopic treatment of submucous fibroids[20] has been a significant therapeutic advance.

The choice of these and other techniques for the investigation of women with fibroids will depend largely on the presenting features of each case, the clinical problem and proposed management. Increased accuracy in delineating the site and nature of individual fibroids should lead to greater understanding of their clinical significance and lead to improved management.

REFERENCES

1. Buttram, V.C. and Reiter, R.C. (1981). Uterine leiomyomata: etiology, symptomatology and management. *Fertil. Steril.*, **36**, 433–45
2. West, C.P., Lumsden, M.A., Lawson, S., Williamson, J. and Baird, D.T. (1987). Shrinkage of uterine fibroids during therapy with goserelin (Zoladex): a luteinizing hormone-releasing hormone agonist administered as a monthly subcutaneous depot. *Fertil. Steril.*, **48**, 45–51
3. Katz, V.L., Dotters, D.J. and Droegemueller, W. (1989). Complications of uterine leiomyomas in pregnancy. *Obstet. Gynecol.*, **73**, 593–6
4. Muram, D., Gillieson, M. and Walters, J.H. (1980). Myomas of the uterus in pregnancy, ultrasonographic follow up. *Am. J. Obstet. Gynecol.*, **138**, 16–19
5. Aharoni, A., Reiter, A., Golan, D., Paltiely, Y. and Sharf, M. (1988). Pattern of growth of uterine leiomyomas during pregnancy. A prospective longitudinal study. *Br. J. Obstet. Gynaecol.*, **95**, 510–13
6. Weiss, D.B., Aldor, A. and Aboulafia, Y. (1975). Erythrocytosis due to erythropoeitin-producing uterine fibromyoma. *Am. J. Obstet. Gynecol.*, **122**, 358–60
7. Persaud, V. and Arjoon, P.D. (1970). Uterine leiomyomata: incidence of degenerative change and correlation of associated symptoms. *Obstet. Gynecol.*, **35**, 432–6
8. Vollenhoven, B.J., Lawrence, A.S. and Healy, D. (1990). Uterine fibroids: a clinical review. *Br. J. Obstet. Gynaecol.*, **97**, 285–98
9. Corscaden, J.A. and Singh, B.P. (1958). Leiomyosarcoma of the uterus. *Am. J. Obstet. Gynecol.*, **75**, 149–53
10. Harper, R.S. and Scully, R.E. (1961). Intravenous leiomyomatosis of the

uterus. *Obstet. Gynecol.*, **18**, 519–52

11. Williams, I.A. and Shaw, R.W. (1990). Effect of Nafarelin on uterine fibroids measured by ultrasound and magnetic resonance imaging. *Eur. J. Obstet. Gynecol. Reprod. Biol.*, **34**, 111–17
12. Cochrane, W.J. and Thomas, M.A. (1974). Ultrasound diagnosis of gynaecologic pelvic masses. *Radiology*, **110**, 649–54
13. Levi, S. and Delval, R. (1976). Value of ultrasonic diagnosis of gynaecological tumors in 370 surgical cases. *Acta Obstet. Gynecol. Scand.*, **55**, 261–6
14. Lawson, T.L. and Albarelli, J.N. (1977). Diagnosis of gynecologic pelvic masses by gray scale ultrasonography: analysis of specificity and accuracy. *Am. J. Roentgenol.*, **128**, 1003–6
15. Walsh, J.W., Taylor, K.J.W., Wasson, J.F. McL., Schwartz, P.E. and Rosenfield, A. (1979). Gray scale ultrasound in 204 proven gynaecological masses: accuracy and specific diagnostic criteria. *Radiology*, **130**, 391–7
16. West, C.P. and Lumsden, M.A. (1989). Fibroids and menorrhagia. In Drife, J. (ed.) *Dysfunctional Uterine Bleeding and Menorrhagia, – Baillière's Clinical Obstetrics and Gynaecology*, Vol. 3, pp. 357–74. (London: Balliere)
17. Hricak, H., Tscholakoff, D., Heinrichs, L., Fisher, M.R., Dooms, G.C., Reinhold, C. and Jaffe, R.B. (1986). Uterine leiomyomas: correlation of MR, histopathologic findings and symptoms. *Radiology*, **158**, 385–91
18. Maheux, R., Lemay, A., Blanchet, P., Friede, J. and Pratt, X. (1991). Maintained reduction of uterine leiomyoma following addition of hormonal replacement therapy to a monthly luteinizing hormone-releasing hormone agonist implant: a pilot study. *Hum. Reprod.* **6**, 500–5
19. Gimpleson, R.J. and Rappold, H.O. (1988). A comparative study between panoramic hysteroscopy with directed biopsy and dilatation and curettage. *Am. J. Obstet. Gynecol.*, **158**, 489–92
20. Siegler, A.M. and Valle, R.F. (1988). Therapeutic hysteroscopic procedures. *Fertil. Steril.*, **50**, 685–701

5

Fibroids and infertility

P. Vercellini, L. Bocciolone, M.T. Rognoni and G. Bolis

INTRODUCTION

That fibroids may complicate the course of pregnancy and delivery is an old and undisputed clinical tenet. The relation between fibroids and infertility is much more uncertain. Given the high prevalence of these tumours in women of reproductive age, it is not surprising to find that a significant proportion of women attempting to conceive are affected. Any delay in conception causes anxiety in the couple and 'obliges' the gynaecologist to find an explanation and propose a treatment. According to the traditional canons of anatomy and pathology, a fibroid is an anomaly. The presence of a fibroid provides the gynaecologist with a reason for the couple's failure to conceive, thus avoiding the frustrations of a 'diagnosis' of unexplained infertility. A spate of hypotheses, some probable and others less so, have been proposed to explain how fibroids may prevent conception. Once the pathogenesis of the symptom has been hypothesized, the logical process continues cascade-fashion through the stages of diagnosis, classification and treatment, although the prevalence of the presumed disease in the healthy population has not been ascertained, and whether the anomaly is really the cause of the symptom is still unknown. In this paper the recent literature is analysed in an attempt to throw light on these last two points.

EPIDEMIOLOGICAL DATA

Fibroids are the commonest tumours found in women, occurring in 20–25% of the female population over the age of 30[1]. Growth of these neoplasms is generally slow, so their clinical recognition rises markedly during the fourth decade of life. Furthermore, the current trend of postponing childbearing[2] may increase the prevalence of fibroids among women desiring offspring, artificially raising the incidence of infertility associated with the tumour. Estimates of its prevalence are mainly based on findings at pelvic exploration. However, the increasingly frequent use of ultrasonography, especially with the transvaginal probe[3], and of sophisticated methods like magnetic resonance imaging[4], could increase the estimated prevalence of myomas appreciably, due to accurate diagnosis of tumours which are not detectable clinically. Moreover, these methods could reveal a higher prevalence than expected, also earlier in reproductive age. The consequences of the increased recognition of small fibroids are difficult to predict, but, for example, the recognition of minimal, subtle, atypical and non-pigmented endometriotic lesions has recently assumed great importance in infertile women.

There are few population-based data on fibroids. Clinical data are derived from selected series composed mainly of women with fibroids who have symptoms that require medical intervention. The variability in symptoms in relation to site and volume of the tumours is well known and impressive.

Ross and colleagues[5], analysing data from the Oxford Family Planning Association cohort study, found an inverse relationship between the number of term pregnancies and the occurrence of fibroids. However, they concluded that relative infertility seems unlikely to be the whole explanation, because absolute infertility was uncommon (89% (478) of the women with fibroids had had at least one term pregnancy). Furthermore, contraceptive use after study entry was only slightly and not significantly less in the fibroid group, compared to the controls (average duration of contraceptive use: 69.4 versus 71.3 months). Also, the interval between marriage and first birth was only slightly different in the two groups (relative risk of 1.20 for ≥ 10 years versus < 2 years). In addition, the authors observed that the relative risk for fibroids was slightly but not significantly increased in association with miscarriage. In a case–control study performed in the greater Milan area[6], based on 275 operated women with histologically confirmed fibroids and 722 controls with acute non-gynaecological or hormone-related conditions, no association was found between the number of spontaneous abortions and the tumour. Interestingly, the reported protective effect of pregnancy on the risk of development and growth of fibroids does not seem to apply to preoperative term pregnancies in patients undergoing myomectomy, since being parous or nulliparous at surgery did not affect the risk of recurrence in a large consecutive series studied at the Department of Obstetrics and Gynaecology of the University of Milan[7]. This could be explained, in part, by a more frequent use of combined oral contraceptives, which seem to diminish the risk of fibroids in parous women[5,8].

HOW COULD FIBROIDS CAUSE INFERTILITY?

Numerous theories have been advanced to explain how fibroids cause infertility. An association with anovulation has been suggested[9]. This would be supported by the reported elevated incidence of endometrial abnormalities, ranging from atrophy to hyperplasia, found concomitantly with fibroids[10]. However, no study has demonstrated conclusively that the incidence of anovulation is higher in women with fibroids than controls. The normal ovulatory cycles observed in most women with fibroids argues against anovulation as the primary cause of infertility[11].

Large leiomyomas may interfere with the passage of sperm by distorting the endometrial cavity or by interfering with uterine contractions which may facilitate sperm transport[12,13]. Cervical fibroids may compress the cervical canal or alter the position of the cervix, thereby interfering with sperm capture in the posterior fornix[12,14]. Cornual myomas may impinge on the tubal lumina and distort the course of the Fallopian tube. Gardner and Shaw[15] used gonadotropin releasing hormone (GnRH) agonists to treat patients with intramural occlusion by cornual myomas; tubal patency was restored as shown by hysterosalpingography, and pregnancy was achieved. Impairment of nidation and implantation may be due to one or more factors including endometrial atrophy or ulceration resulting from submucous tumours[16], increased myometrial irritability and contractility[17], degenerative changes within the leiomyomas, and endometrial vascular changes caused by compression and obstruction of endometrial and myometrial vessels. According to the radiographic data of Farrer-Brown and co-workers[18], by causing venous dilatation and congestion or impairment of blood flow, impingement on endometrial and myometrial venous plexi may alter the endometrial environment in such a way that proper nidation of the fertilized egg is prevented. This possibility is supported by Forssman's observation[19] that blood flow, as determined by locally injected xenon, is lower in fibroids and adjacent tissues than in normal uteri. Some of the above causes have been proposed also to explain the reported elevated incidence of miscarriage in women with fibroids.

DO FIBROIDS REALLY CAUSE INFERTILITY?

Whether fibroids are a causal factor of infertility remains controversial. Because of their ubiquity among women of reproductive age, the mere presence of these tumours may not necessarily be responsible for impaired reproductive function. Although 27–40% of women with multiple leiomyomas are infertile, other causes of infertility are present in the majority of such patients[14]. In a series of 677 women undergoing surgery for infertility, Buttram and Reiter[20] found that only 1.8% of the Caucasian patients had infertility attributable to leiomyomas alone. They concluded that whereas infertility is frequently associated with myomas that necessitate surgery, the tumours do not contribute significantly to the overall incidence of infertility. The conviction that myomas cause infertility derives mostly from results of observational studies in which slightly over half of the patients who underwent conservative surgery subsequently conceived (Table 1). However, few authors have performed myomectomy only on subjects with otherwise unexplained infertility and none of the studies published so far was controlled. Indeed, no studies have mentioned the number of patients with significant fibroids who have had term deliveries.

Recently, Wheeler and Malinak[32,33] applied the criteria of Sackett and colleagues[34] for causality to the literature data on endometriosis in order to analyse the association between the disease and infertility. The same nine diagnostic tests for causation may be applied to data on fibroids (Table 2).

The first criterion is the experimental evidence in humans. Sackett and colleagues[34] state that this criterion is met only if randomized experimental trials confirm the proposed causal relation. There are no such data on the supposed fibroids-associated infertility. The second criterion

Table 1 Post-myomectomy pregnancy rates according to the literature

Authors and year	*Modality*	*Number operated*	*Number wanting children*	*Number conceiving*	*(%)*
Loeffler and Noble[21], 1970	Laparotomy	180	23	9	(39)
Babaknia *et al.*[22], 1978	Laparotomy	46	46	22	(48)
Ranney and Frederick[23], 1979	Laparotomy	51	9	8	(89)
Buttram and Reiter[20], 1981	Laparotomy	59	10	5	(50)
Berkeley *et al.*[24], 1983	Laparotomy	50	50	25	(50)
Garcia and Tureck[16], 1984	Laparotomy	17	15	8	(53)
Rosenfeld[25], 1986	Laparotomy	23	23	15	(65)
Hallez *et al.*[26], 1987	Hysteroscopy	61	11	7	(64)
Starks[27], 1988	Laparotomy	32	32	20	(63)
Brooks *et al.*[28], 1989	Hysteroscopy	79	13	4	(31)
Smith and Uhlir[29], 1990	Laparotomy	63	32	16	(50)
Donnez *et al.*[30], 1990	Hysteroscopy	60	24	16	(66)
Corson and Brooks[31], 1991	Hysteroscopy	92	13	10	(77)
Total		856	314	172	(55)

Table 2 Satisfaction of the nine diagnostic tests of Sackett *et al.*[34] for causation according to the current literature on fibroids; the tests are listed in decreasing order of importance in proving causation (as adapted by Wheeler and Malinak[32,33])

Diagnostic tests	*Does current literature demonstrate that fibroids cause infertility?*
1. Is there experimental evidence from human studies?	No
2. Is the association strong?	No
3. Is the association consistent from study to study?	No
4. Is the temporal relation correct?	No
5. Is there a dose–response gradient?	No
6. Does the association make epidemiological sense?	Yes
7. Does the association make biological sense?	Yes/No
8. Is the association specific?	No
9. Is the association analogous to a previously proven causal association?	No

concerns the strength of the proposed association. Apart from the lack of controls without fibroids in published studies, the weakness of the association is clinically and epidemiologically evident. This leads to a negative answer to the third criterion because, indeed, it is consistently reported that fibroids do not always cause infertility. With regard to the fourth test, the temporal relation between myomas and infertility cannot be established. A prospective study would be needed that used transvaginal ultrasonography, hysteroscopy or magnetic resonance imaging to investigate asymptomatic women and identify a group who first develop fibroids and then later complain of infertility. This seems impractical. The fifth criterion, a dose–response curve, is not met since clinical data demonstrate that there is no such close relationship between the number and size of fibroids and the probability of conception. The answer to the sixth criterion is positive since fibroids and infertility coexist in the same population of reproductive-age women. The seventh criterion is only partly met. In fact, although on one hand the association between infertility and submucous or cornual myomas makes biological sense, there is no reason why subserous fibroids should prevent conception. The answer to the eighth criterion on specificity must be no, since infertility has many other causes. Neither is the ninth criterion met, since fibroids – especially if small and/or subserous – may be considered like limited endometriotic lesions and circumscribed pelvic adhesions, and it has still not been possible to prove that these conditions have a causal relationship with infertility[35–37].

Can it be claimed with certainty, at this point, that fibroids do not have any role in determining infertility? Obviously the response to this question is also no. Probably, fibroids are simply a heterogeneous group of tumours which, in some particular situations, make conception unlikely although in most cases they constitute an occasional finding in infertility workups. In this regard, it is curious that the American Fertility Society, which has classified many disorders associated with infertility including endometriosis, adnexal adhesions, tubal occlusions, tubal pregnancies, Müllerian anomalies and intrauterine adhesions[38,39] has still not classified uterine leiomyomas. It is not clear whether a classification has been judged neither useful nor necessary, in this case, or whether fibroids are not considered an important cause of infertility.

Similarly, the reported association between miscarriage and fibroids seems uncertain. In one review of several large series totalling 1941 patients, the miscarriage rate was 41% preoperatively and 19% after myomectomy[20]. The question that arises here is what would have happened if these women had attempted another pregnancy without undergoing surgery. We know, in fact, that in most single miscarriages the cause is genetic and that for habitual abortions there is a massive placebo effect related to the simple psychological support provided by the obstetric team[40]. A quotation from an authoritative text such as *Williams Obstetrics*[41] is particularly relevant in this regard:

> 'Even large and multiple uterine leiomyomas are not usually associated with abortion, and their location apparently is more important than size. Submucous, but not intramural or subserous myomas are more likely to cause abortion. Even so, leiomyomas should be regarded as a causative factor only if the remainder of the clinical investigation is negative and a hysterogram shows a filling defect in the endometrial cavity. Myomectomies to remove such tumours often result in a scarred uterus which may rupture during a subsequent pregnancy either before or during labor. The only certain method to assess the possibility that a leiomyoma might be associated with abortion is to allow pregnancy'.

CONCLUSIONS

(1) Epidemiological data reveal a higher frequency of nulliparity among subjects with fibroids, compared to controls. This confirms the protective effect of term pregnancies, but does not prove a definite relation between reproductive problems and fibroids. The suggested association between these tumours and miscarriage does not seem to be substantiated.

(2) Fibroids may cause infertility when they distort the endometrial cavity or occlude the intramural portion of the tubes. In other situations they have no proven causal role in impeding conception. The proposal that intramural and submucous tumours of ≥2 cm, subserous tumours that may be large enough to encroach upon a tubal lumen or adjacent structures, and pedunculated submucous myomas of any size should be removed in women with otherwise unexplained infertility[20], seems acceptable for now.

(3) Further epidemiological studies and randomized, controlled clinical trials relating results to site, volume and number of fibroids might eventually clarify whether there is a causal relation between fibroids and infertility or merely a chance association.

REFERENCES

1. Vollenhoven, B.J., Lawrence, A.S. and Healy, D.L. (1990). Uterine fibroids: a clinical review. *Br. J. Obstet. Gynaecol.*, **97**, 285–98
2. Holloway, S. and Brock, D.J.H. (1988). Changes in maternal age distribution and their possible impact on demand for prenatal diagnostic services. *Br. Med. J.*, **296**, 978–81
3. Fedele, L., Bianchi, S., Dorta, M., Brioschi, D., Zanotti, F. and Vercellini, P. (1991). Transvaginal ultrasonography versus hysteroscopy in the diagnosis of uterine submucous myomas. *Obstet. Gynecol.*, **77**, 745–8
4. Dudiak, C.M., Turner, D.A., Patel, S.K., Archie, J.T., Silver, B. and Norusis, M. (1988). Uterine leiomyomas in the infertile patient: preoperative localization with MR imaging versus US and hysterosalpingography. *Radiology*, **167**, 627–30
5. Ross, R.K., Pike, M.C., Vessey, M.P., Bull, D., Yeates, D. and Casagrande, J.T. (1986). Risk factors for uterine fibroids: reduced risk associated with oral contraceptives. *Br. Med. J.*, **293**, 359–62
6. Parazzini, F., La Vecchia, C., Negri, E., Cecchetti, G. and Fedele, L. (1988). Epidemiologic characteristics of women with uterine fibroids: a case–control study. *Obstet. Gynecol.*, **72**, 853–7
7. Candiani, G.B., Fedele, L., Parazzini, F. and Villa, L. (1991). Risk of recurrence after myomectomy. *Br. J. Obstet. Gynaecol.*, **98**, 385–9
8. Anonymous (1991). Recurrence of fibroids after myomectomy. *Lancet*, **338**, 548
9. Miller, N.F., Ludovici, P.P. and Arbor, A. (1955). On the origin and development of uterine fibroids. *Am. J. Obstet. Gynecol.*, **70**, 720–40
10. Deligdish, L. and Loewenthal, M. (1970). Endometrial changes associated with myomata of the uterus. *J. Clin. Pathol.*, **23**, 676–80
11. Buttram, V.C. and Reiter, R.C. (1985). Uterine leiomyomata. In Buttram, V.C. and Reiter, R.C. (eds.) *Surgical Treatment of the Infertile Female*, pp.201–28. (Baltimore: Williams & Wilkins)
12. Hunt, J.E. and Wallach, E.E. (1974). Uterine factors in infertility – an overview. *Clin. Obstet. Gynecol.*, **17**, 44–64
13. Clement, P.B. (1991). Pathology of gamete and zygote transport: cervical, endometrial, myometrial, and tubal factors in infertility. In Kraus, F.T.,

Damjanov, I. and Kaufman, N. (eds.) *Pathology of Reproductive Failure*, pp.140–94. (Baltimore: Williams & Wilkins)

14. Rubin, I.C. (1958). Uterine fibromyomas and sterility. *Clin. Obstet. Gynecol.*, **1**, 501–33
15. Gardner, R.L. and Shaw, R.W. (1989). Cornual fibroids: a conservative approach to restoring tubal patency using a gonadotropin-releasing hormone agonist (goserelin) with successful pregnancy. *Fertil. Steril.*, **52**, 332–4
16. Garcia, C.R. and Tureck, R.W. (1984). Submucosal leiomyomas and infertility. *Fertil. Steril.*, **42**, 16–19
17. Huszar, G. and Walsh, M.P. (1989). Biochemistry of the myometrium and cervix. In Wynn, R.M. and Jollie, W.P. (eds.) *Biology of the Uterus*, 2nd edn., pp.355–402. (New York: Plenum Medical Book Co.)
18. Farrer-Brown, G., Beilby, J.O.W. and Tarbit, M.H. (1971). Venous changes in the endometrium of myomatous uteri. *Obstet. Gynecol.*, **38**, 743–51
19. Forssman, L. (1976). Distribution of blood flow in myomatous uteri as measured by locally-injected 133 Xenon. *Acta Obstet. Gynecol. Scand.*, **55**, 101–6
20. Buttram, V.C. and Reiter, R.C. (1981). Uterine leiomyomata: Etiology, symptomatology and management. *Fertil. Steril.*, **36**, 433–55
21. Loeffler, F.E. and Noble, A.D. (1970). Myomectomy at the Chelsea Hospital for women. *J. Obstet. Gynecol. Br. Commonw.*, **77**, 167–71
22. Babaknia, A., Rock, J.A. and Jones, H.W. (1978). Pregnancy success following abdominal myomectomy for infertility. *Fertil. Steril.*, **30**, 644–7
23. Ranney, B. and Frederick, I. (1979). The occasional need for myomectomy. *Obstet. Gynecol.*, **53**, 437–42
24. Berkeley, A.S., DeCherney, A.D. and Polan, M.L. (1983). Abdominal myomectomy and subsequent fertility. *Surg. Gynecol. Obstet.*, **156**, 319–22
25. Rosenfeld, D.L. (1986). Abdominal myomectomy for otherwise unexplained infertility. *Fertil. Steril.*, **46**, 328–30
26. Hallez, J.P., Netter, A. and Cartier, R. (1987). Methodical intrauterine resection. *Am. J. Obstet. Gynecol.*, **156**, 1080–4
27. Starks, G.C. (1988). CO_2 laser myomectomy in an infertile population. *J. Reprod. Med.*, **33**, 184–6
28. Brooks, P.G., Loffer, F.D. and Serden, S.P. (1989). Resectoscopic removal of symptomatic intrauterine lesions. *J. Reprod. Med.*, **34**, 435–7
29. Smith, D.C. and Uhlir, J.K. (1990). Myomectomy as a reproductive procedure. *Am. J. Obstet. Gynecol.*, **162**, 1476–82
30. Donnez, J., Gillerot, S., Bourgonjon, D., Clerckx, F. and Nisolle, M. (1990). Neodymium:YAG laser hysteroscopy in large submucous fibroids. *Fertil. Steril.*, **54**, 999–1003

31. Corson, S.L. and Brooks, P.G. (1991). Resectoscopic myomectomy. *Fertil. Steril.*, **55**, 1041–4
32. Wheeler, J.M. and Malinak, L.R. (1988). Does mild endometriosis cause infertility? *Sem. Reprod. Endocrinol.*, **6**, 239–49
33. Wheeler, J.M. (1989). Epidemiology of endometriosis-associated infertility. *J. Reprod. Med.*, **34**, 41–6
34. Sackett, D.L., Haynes, R.B. and Tugwell, P. (1985). Clinical epidemiology: a basic science for clinical medicine. pp.223–34. (Boston: Little Brown)
35. Candiani, G.B., Vercellini, P., Fedele, L., Nava, S. and Fontana, P.E. (1990). Medical treatment of mild endometriosis associated with infertility. *Eur. J. Obstet. Gynecol.*, **38**, 169–80
36. Candiani, G.B., Vercellini, P., Fedele, L., Bocciolone, L. and Bianchi, S. (1990). Medical treatment of mild endometriosis in infertile women: analysis of a failure. *Hum. Reprod.*, **5** 901–5
37. Candiani, G.B., Vercellini, P., Fedele, L., Colombo, A. and Candiani, M. (1991). Mild endometriosis and infertility: a critical review of epidemiologic data, diagnostic pitfalls, and classification limits. *Obstet. Gynecol. Surv.*, **46**, 374–82
38. The American Fertility Society. (1985). Revised American Fertility Society classification of endometriosis: 1985. *Fertil. Steril.*, **43**, 351–2
39. The American Fertility Society. (1988). The American Fertility Society classifications of adnexal adhesions, distal tubal occlusion, tubal occlusion secondary to tubal ligation, tubal pregnancies, Müllerian anomalies and intrauterine adhesions. *Fertil. Steril.*, **49**, 944–55
40. Stray-Pederson, B. and Stray-Pederson, S. (1984). Etiological factors and subsequent reproductive performance in 195 couples with a prior history of habitual abortion. *Am. J. Obstet. Gynecol.*, **148**, 140–6
41. Cunningham, F.G., MacDonald, P.C. and Gant, N.F. (1989). Complication of pregnancy. In *Williams Obstetrics*, 18th edn., pp.489–777. (Norwalk: Appleton & Lange)

6

Fibroids and menorrhagia

M.A. Lumsden

INTRODUCTION

Uterine leiomyomata (fibroids), are common, benign tumours occurring in about 25% of women over the age of 35 years[1]. They are composed predominantly of smooth muscle with a variable amount of connective tissue and are classified according to their position within the uterus being either submucosal, intramural or subserosal. They are commonly multiple and may cause considerable enlargement and distortion of the uterus.

Fibroids may be asymptomatic or may present with infertility, early pregnancy loss, or menstrual problems associated with or without pelvic discomfort and dysmenorrhoea.

FIBROIDS AND MENORRHAGIA

Fibroids are considered to be a common cause of menorrhagia although the actual proportion associated with heavy menstrual loss is unclear. This uncertainty arises from the fact that menorrhagia in the absence of pathology (dysfunctional uterine bleeding) is common at about the same time of life as fibroids occur and it is difficult to be certain that they are not an incidental finding. In a review of women undergoing myomectomy, 30% of them complained of menorrhagia[2] although the proportion varied from 17 to 62% in the nine different studies described. However, these studies are difficult to interpret since they use a subjective assessment of menstrual blood loss. Measurement of menstrual blood loss is important since about 50% of those complaining of menorrhagia actually have a loss within the normal range. Studies where such measurement has been performed are rare. Rybo and colleagues[3] found that 40% of women with a menstrual blood loss in excess of 200 ml had uterine fibroids whereas only 10% of those with a loss of 80–100 ml were affected. In a further study of 18 women with fibroids, where menstrual blood loss was also measured using the alkaline haematin method, 15 of the women demonstrated genuine menorrhagia (a loss of > 80 ml/period) and the remainder had a loss at the upper limit of normal. Three of the women with losses of over 350 ml/period had intrauterine fibroid polyps and six had a haemoglobin level less than 10 g/dl[4]. These studies suggest a connection between fibroids and heavy menstrual loss, but this assertion has been challenged. Miller and colleagues[5] attributed the symptoms only to the presence of submucous fibroids. The importance of position is discussed further below.

Heavy menstrual loss is the commonest cause of anaemia in the Western world. Fraser and co-workers[4] suggest that anaemia is commoner among those women with menorrhagia associated with fibroids. We have also studied over 100 women with uterine fibroids in detail[6–8] and 12% overall had a haemoglobin level less than 10 g/dl, although of these 15% did not complain of menorrhagia. Unfortunately, we have no objective measurement of blood loss on these patients.

THE IMPORTANCE OF POSITION

Submucous fibroids frequently cause distortion of the uterine cavity (Figure 1) and this is assumed to be the cause of the menstrual problems. In our studies cited above, only 40% of those having hysterectomy to remove a fibroid uterus with the subjective complaint of menorrhagia had submucous fibroids diagnosed at operation. This is in agreement with a small study of women with severe anaemia (haemoglobin levels < 9.5 g/dl) in the presence of fibroids where submucous tumours were present in only seven out of 16 cases (single in three cases and multiple in four)[9]. A report of one South African series states that submucous fibroids were present in only 25% of those with menorrhagia[10] and Novak and Woodruff[11] estimate that 10% of fibroids overall are submucous. It now

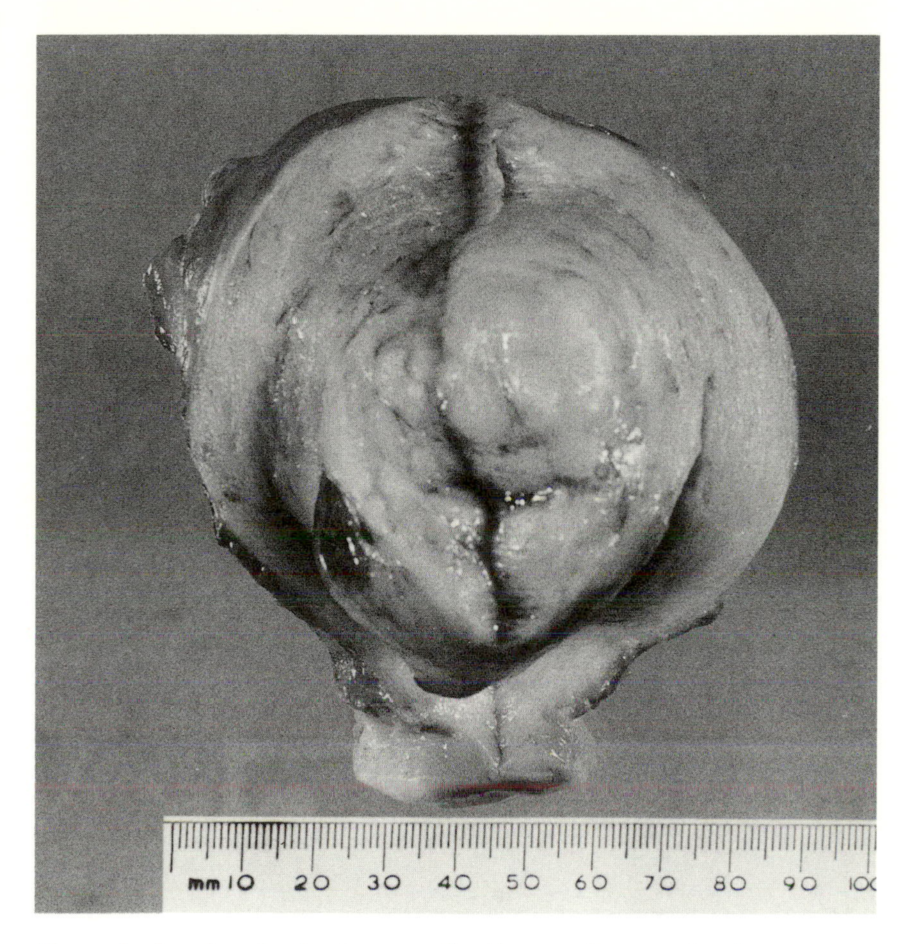

Figure 1 A pedunculated, submucous fibroid removed at operation from a woman suffering from menorrhagia and lower abdominal pain

seems clear that heavy menstrual loss may be associated with fibroids at any site. This is important when considering treatment, which is discussed further below.

AETIOLOGY OF FIBROID-ASSOCIATED MENORRHAGIA

Abnormal endometrial function is thought to be an important factor in the aetiology of dysfunctional uterine bleeding. It is likely that abnormal production of local factors, one of which comprises the prostaglandins[12] contributes to bleeding. Prostaglandins are produced by fibroids[13] and it appears that the metabolite of prostacyclin (6-keto-PGF_1) is produced in amounts similar to those in healthy myometrium, whereas the production of thromboxane B_2 is less[14]. Prostaglandin I_2 is a vasodilator and thromboxane a vasoconstrictor so there is a predominance of the former which may contribute to the heavy menstrual loss. In the study by Fraser and co-workers[4] the presence of prostaglandin synthetase inhibitors resulted in a decreased loss in six out of nine women, although the reduction in blood loss for the whole group was not statistically significant (means $\pm$ SEM before and during treatment were 102.3 ± 13.1 and 88.4 ± 17.1 ml respectively) and was clinically valuable in only three women. These findings suggest that other factors are of more importance.

The increased surface area is thought to be important in the aetiology of menorrhagia although there is no evidence for this. In dysfunctional uterine bleeding, i.e. in the absence of fibroids, the surface area is of no importance and is not related to the menstrual loss[15]. Fibroids may affect the way the uterus contracts but, again, myometrial contraction is not thought to be important in controlling blood loss in the non-pregnant uterus. It is more likely to be important in the aetiology of dysmenorrhoea (see below). Buttram and Reiter[2] have suggested that the fibroids affect the blood flow through the uterus causing pressure on the venous output and the formation of venous lakes. This may help explain why fibroids at all sites may be associated with menorrhagia.

It has also been suggested that menorrhagia associated with fibroids may be due to abnormal uterine contractility[16]. In general, this is not considered to be an important mechanism in the control of the volume of blood lost in the non-pregnant uterus, unlike the pregnant uterus, although it may be very important as a cause of menstrually associated pain. Abnormalities in the pattern of contractility have been demonstrated in dysmenorrhoea in the presence of fibroids[17], these patterns differing from those normally associated with primary dysmenorrhoea[18]. This may reflect the differences in the proportions of smooth muscle and connective tissue in fibroids compared to normal myometrium.

MANAGEMENT

This depends on the severity of the symptoms, and the age and reproductive state of the patient. Where symptoms are present, or the fibroids are very large, intervention is often required. This may be either medical or surgical.

Surgical treatment

If a woman wishes to maintain fertility, then myomectomy is the surgical treatment of choice. This may be performed by laparotomy or, more recently, via the laparoscope or hysteroscope. Removal of the fibroids alone is a good way of assessing the relationship between fibroids and menorrhagia. A survey of the literature suggests that 80% of patients so treated achieve symptomatic relief, which supports the concept that fibroids cause menstrual problems[2]. Further support for this idea comes from a recent study of hysteroscopic myomectomy where the surrounding myometrium was left intact[19]. Menorrhagia was relieved in over 80% of subjects. However, in a small study of hysteroscopic myomectomy where ten women had their fibroids partially removed, (only the portion protruding into the cavity was removed), success was claimed in eight cases, the remaining two requiring conventional myomectomy[20]. If these results are confirmed by larger studies then they are of considerable interest, since it would appear that it is not necessary to remove all the fibroid tissue to relieve menorrhagia. It would also suggest that distortion of the uterine cavity is a vital factor.

For those who have completed their families, the conventional treatment is hysterectomy. Fibroids are a common reason for hysterectomies, accounting for 30% of those performed in the United States and 20% of those in Scotland. The operation may be difficult and preoperative treatment with a gonadotropin releasing hormone (GnRH) agonist which decreases fibroid size may facilitate the procedure[6]. In a recent study, 71 women having hysterectomy for fibroids were randomized to receive either the GnRH agonist goserelin, given as a subcutaneous depot once monthly, or a sham injection. None of the operations in the goserelin group was considered by the surgeon to be technically difficult, compared with six operations in the untreated group. Also, the operative blood loss was significantly less in the treated group (Figure 2). The beneficial effect is likely to be due partly to the decrease in size and partly to the decrease in uterine blood flow induced by the agonist[21]. It is also possible that pretreatment will enable more fibroids to be removed hysteroscopically, but this is discussed in more detail in Chapter 9.

Medical treatment

There is now an increasing demand for treatments which avoid the necessity for surgery. Hysterectomy is accompanied by a small mortality and considerable morbidity[22] and it is not only those who wish to maintain fertility who wish to avoid operation. Various endocrine treatments have been utilized with reasonable success.

Prostaglandin synthetase inhibitors

The treatment of fibroid-associated menorrhagia with this group of drugs has been alluded to above. Overall, there seems to be little benefit, as the small reduction in blood flow achieved is not sufficient to bring those patients with very heavy losses down into the normal range, making these drugs of little use clinically[4,23].

Progestogens

Progestogens have little effect on fibroid size[24,25] and their benefit to those with dysfunctional uterine bleeding alone is uncertain[26]. They are therefore seldom prescribed for fibroid-associated menorrhagia.

Oral contraceptives

The most commonly used oral contraceptive pills contain oestrogen and thus many consider that it should not be prescribed to those with fibroids. There is also a report of fibroid enlargement during oral contraceptive therapy[27]. There is, however, evidence that the pill may protect against later development of fibroids[28] particularly if the formula is high in gestagen.

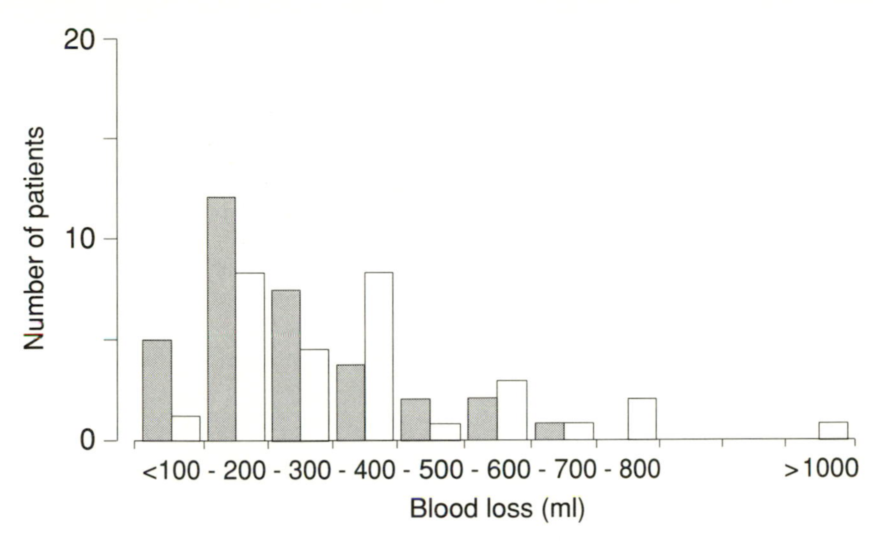

Figure 2 Blood loss at operation (total abdominal hysterectomy) in patients who had received GnRH agonist for 3 months preoperatively (Zoladex®, shaded bars) compared with a second group who received sham depot (clear bars). Excessively heavy blood loss was confined to those receiving sham depot

Androgens

Danazol is frequently used to induce oligomenorrhoea or amenorrhoea in those with DUB (dysfunctional uterine bleeding)[29]. However, there is little published information concerning its use in the presence of fibroids. It has little effect on fibroid size although high doses are likely to induce amenorrhoea as a result of endometrial atrophy and thus relieve the symptoms. Gestrinone is a trienic 19-norsteroid which also relieves symptoms with little alteration in uterine volume[30]. However, side-effects with these preparations are common and short courses are usually preferred.

Gonadotropin releasing hormone agonists

GnRH agonists induce hypo-oestrogenism and a decrease in fibroid size[7,31]. Endometrial atrophy also occurs, leading to amenorrhoea, which is beneficial in anaemic women as a significant rise in haemoglobin occurs[9]. Regrowth of fibroids occurs after cessation of treatment, and in those with dysfunctional uterine bleeding, menorrhagia recurs rapidly[32]. However, in spite of this, a significant number of women claim a 'carry over' benefit of this treatment and many are able to avoid hysterectomy, particularly in the older age-group[33]. GnRH agonists are also of benefit if given prior to hysterectomy, as discussed previously, since operative blood loss is decreased (Figure 2) and the operations are rated as easier by the surgeons involved[6]. The principal disadvantage of the GnRH agonists is the presence of postmenopausal side-effects which occur to some extent in the majority of treated women. This may be relieved partially by the addition of other hormonal preparations. We have studied the effect of goserelin in combination with tamoxifen, since the latter is known to be a partial oestrogen and also has a bone-sparing effect. When given alone, tamoxifen causes a significant increase in ovarian steroid output although there is no consistent increase in gonadotropin release[34,35]. The fibroids either stay the same size or may increase slightly, but because of an antagonist effect at the level of the endometrium, relief of menstrual symptoms commonly occurs[6] (Figure 3). Consequently, even though the fibroids are still present, many of the women are happy with this treatment. When given in combination with goserelin, tamoxifen acts both as agonist and antagonist, in that no fibroid shrinkage occurs. Unfortunately, however, the hot flushes are even worse than on goserelin alone[8]. Medroxyprogesterone acetate (MPA) is also a steroid with a bone-sparing effect[35]. If it is given with goserelin it will prevent fibroid shrinkage, although there is relief of menstrual symptoms and little hot flushing. However, when goserelin is given alone for 3 months and MPA is then added in combination with it, the initial fibroid shrinkage is maintained[37]. We are now performing longer-term studies with this combination in order to increase the clinical usefulness of the agonists.

CONCLUSIONS

In summary, menstrual problems associated with fibroids may be relieved without the necessity of removing the fibroids themselves. This does not mean that the fibroids are unimportant when considering factors causing the menorrhagia, rather that an intact endometrium is necessary for this symptom to occur, and menorrhagia can be relieved without removing the fibroids.

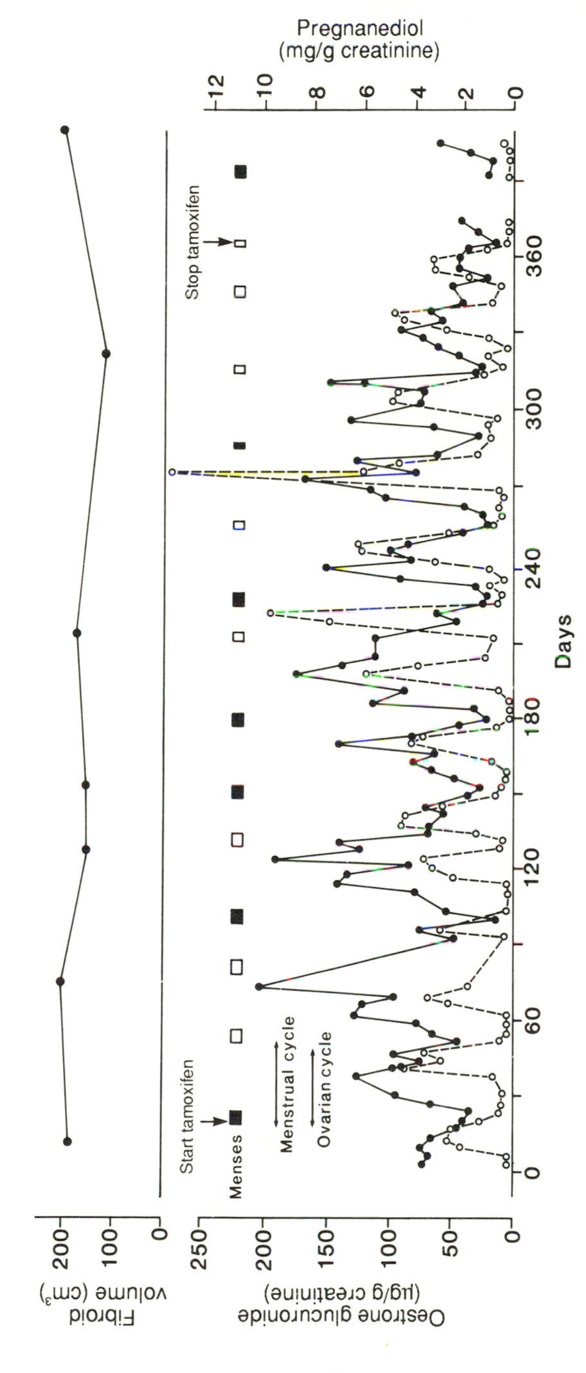

Figure 3 Fibroid size, bleeding pattern and ovarian steroid hormone output (as assessed by measurement of urinary metabolites) of a woman treated with continuous 30 mg tamoxifen daily

REFERENCES

1. Smith, C.J. (1952). Hysterectomy for benign pelvic conditions. *Am. J. Obstet. Gynecol.*, **64**, 1211–20
2. Buttram, V.C. and Reiter, R.C. (1981). Uterine leiomyomata: etiology, symptomatology and management. *Fertil. Steril.*, **36**, 433–45
3. Rybo, G., Leman, J. and Tibbin, R. (1985). Epidemiology of menstrual blood loss. In Baird, D.T. and Michie, E.A. (eds.) *Mechanisms of Menstrual Bleeding*, pp.181–93. (New York: Raven Press)
4. Fraser, I., McCarron, G., Markham, R., Resta, T. and Watts, A. (1986). Measured menstrual loss in women with menorrhagia associated with pelvic disease or coagulation disorder. *Obstet. Gynecol.*, **68**, 630–3
5. Miller, N.F., Ludovici, P.P. and Dontas, E. (1953). The problem of the uterine fibroid. *Am. J. Obstet. Gynecol.*, **66**, 734–46
6. Lumsden, M.A., West, C.P. and Baird, D.T. (1987). Goserelin therapy before surgery for uterine fibroids. *Lancet*, **1**, 36–7
7. West, C.P., Lumsden, M.A., Lawson, S., Williamson, J. and Baird, D.T. (1987). Shrinkage of uterine fibroids during therapy with goserelin (Zoladex): a luteinizing hormone-releasing hormone agonist administered as a monthly subcutaneous depot. *Fertil. Steril.*, **48**, 45–51
8. Lumsden, M.A., West, C.P., Hillier, H. and Baird, D.T. (1989). Tamoxifen acts as an oestrogen agonist in women treated with LHRH agonist (Zoladex) and prevents shrinkage of uterine fibroids. *Fertil. Steril.*, **52**, 924–9
9. Candiani, G.B., Vercellini, P., Fedele, L., Arcani, L., Bianchi, S. and Candiani, M. (1990). Use of goserelin depot, a gonadotropin-releasing hormone agonist, for the treatment of menorrhagia and severe anaemia in women with leiomyomata uteri. *Acta Obstet. Gynecol. Scand.*, **69**, 413–15
10. Rubin, A. and Ford, J.A. (1974). Uterine fibromyomata in urban blacks. *S. Afr. Med. J.*, **48**, 2060–3
11. Novak, E.R. and Woodruff, J.D. (1979). Myomas and other benign tumours of the uterus. In Novak, E.R. and Woodruff, J.D. (eds.) *Gynecologic and Obstetric Pathology*, 8th edn., p.260. (Philadelphia: W.B. Saunders)
12. Smith, S.K., Abel, M.H., Kelly, R.W. and Baird, D.T. (1981). Prostaglandin synthesis in the endometrium of women with ovular dysfunctional uterine bleeding. *Br. J. Obstet. Gynaecol.*, **88**, 434–42
13. Rees, M.C. and Turnbull, A. (1985). Leiomyomas release prostaglandins. *Prost. Leuk. Med.*, **18**, 65–8
14. Aitakallio, T. and Tallberg, A. (1990). Prostaglandin and thromboxane synthesis by endometrial cancer and leiomyomas. *Prostaglandins*, **39**, 259–66

15. Chimbira, T.H., Anderson, A.B.M. and Turnbull, A.C. (1980). Relation between measured menstrual blood loss and patient's subjective assessment of loss, duration of bleeding, number of sanitary towels used, uterine weight and endometrial surface area. *Br. J. Obstet. Gynaecol.*, **87**, 603–7
16. Farrer-Brown, G., Beilby, J.O.W. and Tarbit, M.H. (1971). Venous changes in the endometrium of myomatous uteri. *Obstet. Gynecol.*, **38**, 743–51
17. Iosof, C.S. and Akerlund, M. (1983). Fibromyomas and uterine activity. *Acta Obstet. Gynecol. Scand.*, **62**, 165–7
18. Lumsden, M.A. and Baird, D.T. (1985). Intrauterine pressure in dysmenorrhoea. *Acta Obstet. Gynecol. Scand.*, **64**, 183–6
19. Derman, S.G., Rehnstrom, J. and Neuwirth, R.S. (1991). The long-term effectiveness of hysteroscopic treatment of menorrhagia and leiomyomas. *Obstet. Gynecol.*, **77**, 591–4
20. Michlewitz, H. and Reindollar, R.H. (1988). Hysteroscopic myomectomy using hysteroscopic guidance. *Proceedings of the XII World Congress of Gynaecology and Obstetrics*, Rio de Janeiro, abstr. p.661
21. Matta, W.H., Stabile, I., Shaw, R.W. and Campbell, S. (1988). Doppler assessment of uterine blood flow changes in patients with fibroids receiving the gonadotropin-releasing hormone agonist buserelin. *Fertil. Steril.*, **70**, 720–39
22. Dicker, R.C., Greenspan, J.R., Strauss, L.T. *et al.* (1982). Complications of abdominal and vaginal hysterectomy, among women of reproductive age in the United States. *Am. J. Obstet. Gynecol.*, **144**, 841–8
23. Ylikorkala, O. and Pekonen, F. (1986). Naproxen reduces idiopathic but not fibromyomata-induced menorrhagia. *Obstet. Gynecol.*, **68**, 10–12
24. Goodman, A.L. (1946). Progesterone therapy in uterine fibromyomata. *J. Clin. Endocrinol. Metab.*, **6**, 402–8
25. Goldzieher, J.W., Maqueo, M., Aguilar, J.A. and Canales, E. (1966). Induction of degenerative changes in uterine myomas by high dose progestin therapy. *Am. J. Obstet. Gynecol.*, **96**, 1078–87
26. Cameron, I.T., Haining, R., Lumsden, M.A., Reid Thomas, V. and Smith, S.K. (1990). The effects of mefanamic acid and norethisterone on measured menstrual blood loss. *Obstet. Gynecol.*, **76**, 85–8
27. John, A.H. and Martin, R. (1971). Growth of leiomyomata with oestrogen-progesterone therapy. *J. Reprod. Med.*, **6**, 56–8
28. Ross, R.K., Pike, M.C., Vessey, M.P., Bull, D., Yeates, D. and Casagrande, J.T. (1986). Risk factors for uterine fibroids: reduced risk associated with oral contraceptives. *Br. Med. J.*, **293**, 359–62
29. Chimbira, T.H., Cope, E., Anderson, A.B.M. and Bolton, F.G. (1979). The effect of danazol on menorrhagia, coagulation mechanisms,

haematological indices and body weight. *Br. J. Obstet. Gynaecol.*, **86**, 46–50

30. Coutinho, E.M., Boulanger, G.A. and Goncalves, M.T. (1986). Regression of leiomyomata after treatment with gestrinone, an antiestrogen, antiprogesterone. *Am. J. Obstet. Gynecol.*, **155**, 761–7
31. Filicori, M., Hall, D.A., Loughlin, J.S., Rivier, J., Vale, W. and Crowley, W.F. (1983). A conservative approach to the management of uterine leiomyomata: pituitary desensitisation by a luteinizing hormone-releasing hormone analogue. *Am. J. Obstet. Gynecol.*, **147**, 726–7
32. Shaw, R.W. and Fraser, H.M. (1984). Use of a superactive luteinizing hormone-releasing hormone (LHRH) agonist in the treatment of menorrhagia. *Br. J. Obstet. Gynaecol.*, **91**, 913–6
33. West, C.P., Lumsden, M.A. and Baird, J.T. (1992). Goserelin (Zoladex®) in the treatment of fibroids. *Br. J. Obstet. Gynaecol.*, **99** (suppl. 7), 27–30
34. Ricciardi, I. and Ianniruberto, A. (1979). Tamoxifen-induced regression of benign breast lesions. *Obstet. Gynecol.*, **54**, 80–4
35. Lumsden, M.A., West, C.P. and Baird, D.T. (1989). Tamoxifen prolongs the luteal phase in premenopausal women but has no effect on the size of uterine fibroids. *Clin. Endocrinol.*, **31**, 335–43
36. Mandel, F.P., Davidson, B.J., Erlik, Y., Judd, H.L. and Meldrum, D.R. (1982). Effects of progestins on bone metabolism in postmenopausal women. *J. Reprod. Med.*, **27**, 511–14
37. Friedman, A.J., Barbieri, R.L., Doubilet, P.M., Fine, C. and Schiff, I. (1988). A randomised double-blind trial of gonadotropin releasing hormone agonist (leuprolide) with or without medroxy-progesterone acetate in the treatment of leiomyomata uteri. *Fertil. Steril.*, **49**, 404–9

7

Hysterectomy and myomectomy: techniques and risk factors

D.H. Barlow

INTRODUCTION

This symposium is timely in that it reviews the subject of uterine fibroids when we are on the brink of what may well be a new era in the clinical management of this common problem. The introduction of gonadotropin releasing hormone (GnRH) agonist analogues to shrink fibroids, and the development of intrauterine and intra-abdominal endoscopic fibroid resection, are likely to change patterns of management which have been standardized for several decades. These well-established approaches to the management of fibroids can be summarized as:

(1) Palliation by control of symptoms;

(2) Myomectomy where fertility is to be retained; and

(3) Hysterectomy.

The techniques of myomectomy and hysterectomy for fibroids are part of the surgical inheritance of all gynaecologists and form a fundamental aspect of the skills essential for everyday practice in the operating theatre. I propose in this chapter to avoid a step-by-step account of these operative techniques and instead give an account of how our profession arrived at these operative solutions which have served us so well for about half a century. I hope that this approach may demonstrate the continuum of surgical development so that we may view the new approaches as further logical steps in a long process of innovation. Those who wish a blow by blow account of the surgical steps involved in these operations should consult a gynaecological surgery textbook[1].

SURGICAL ORIGINS

I have taken as my starting point the start of the surgical era with the 1866 *Textbook of Uterine Surgery* by the pioneer gynaecologist Dr J. Marian Sims, who spent some years in practice in London[2]. In common with many medical writers of the last century he communicates through personal comment and anecdotal case histories, but at the same time does attempt scientific analysis of the accumulated experience. It is very readable.

Uterine fibroids were viewed as a major clinical problem in gynaecology, but only where the effects on menstruation or adjacent organs were very serious was surgery attempted. Sims tells of a series of '100 virgins consulting for some uterine disease' of whom '24 had fibroid tumours, or one in 4⅙', and in a series of 505 who were 'married and sterile', 95 had fibroid tumours. Overall, 14 were pedunculated, 46 sessile, 53 intramural, three intrauterine, one attached to the sacrum, and two were on the posterior lip of the cervix. Most were large or very large.

He encouraged the use of the uterine probe, recently introduced by Dr Simpson. 'Twenty years ago how few of us could tell whether the uterus was anteverted or retroverted; whether its enlargement, if any, depended upon a mere hypertrophy of its proper tissue, or upon some adventitious growth either within, upon, or near the organ. Now, however, we diagnose uterine complications with the utmost precision – and all by the touch, the tent, and the probe.' One woman 'had been treated by distinguished professors in four of our largest cities and all, without exception, told her she had retroversion. On making an examination, I found the opposite state of things, viz., a complete anteversion, with a tumour filling up the Douglas cul de sac'. Where the sound was unable to pass an acute bend in the uterine cavity a gum elastic bougie could be used. If digital exploration of the uterine cavity was necessary, then there would be pretreatment using a sponge tent to dilate the cervical canal.

The treatment options were limited. Dr Savage of the Samaritan Hospital dilated the cervix using a tent then injected the cavity with a solution of iodine which 'invariably stops the bleeding' and is repeated with each period. Sims described cervical dilation and the puncture and 2-inch incision of a fibroid using a trochar. The fibroid discharged cystic matter and haemorrhage was arrested using 'liquor ferri persulphatis'. The woman was allowed home after 2 months but later her 'abdomen was seemingly as large as ever'. Dr Atlee used enucleation of the whole mass and Dr Baker Brown preferred to gouge the tumour, removing part of it. Sims tried both methods and both women died. Enucleation involved a sequence of steps. Firstly the cervix was incised 'wide open'. The profuse haemorrhage was checked and the tissues allowed to heal. Then the capsule of the fibroid was incised via the uterine cavity and haemorrhage stemmed by tampon. The patient was then 'returned to the country' to await 'the efforts of nature in forcing the tumour down through the artificial opening made in its capsule'. After 3 months there was tumour projecting into the vagina and its attachments were further incised. Six months later she was still having severe haemorrhages and the tumour was now filling the vagina and continuing to grow. A cord was passed around its neck and it was severed under chloroform. The haemorrhage was 'fearful' and she died a few hours later.

Sims argued that, with the exception of the polypoid submucous fibroid whose removal was straightforward, surgery for fibroids should only be undertaken where they 'endanger life'. He did not advocate surgery for the alleviation of sterility unless there were very exceptional circumstances: 'Suppose a dynasty was threatened with extinction, and the cause of sterility was ascertained to be an enucleable fibroid: here the perpetuity of a good government and the welfare of the state might depend upon the result. Would such an operation be justifiable, if the parties, knowing the risks, were willing to assume the responsibilities?'

In his lectures on gynaecology, Dr Atthill of the Rotunda Hospital, Dublin[3] demonstrated that by 1883 methods had further developed. Fibroid polypi could be removed using a 'galvanic knife' which was a loop of platinum wire connected to a battery as a form of cutting cautery. Ergot was now used in the control of haemorrhages. Surgery was used where the patient was likely to die despite the ergot combined with iron and the plugging of the vagina.

Dr Atthill describes a wider range of options than those available in 1866. The cervix could be incised to encourage expulsion of the tumour and an improvement in haemorrhages and pain. The tumour could be incised via the uterine cavity in the hope of decreasing its vitality. This method was unreliable and could be combined with a gouging procedure.

Enucleation remained an option, with division of the capsule and gradual expulsion. Dr Matthews Duncan advocated avulsion which could be used where spontaneous enucleation had begun or where surgical enucleation had been only partially successful. Dr Atthill described an avulsion case who was a 40-year-old widow, and on whom enucleation had been previously carried out. On day 1 the cervix was divided with scissors under chloroform with no significant haemorrhage. She was given oral ergot and 'feri perchoridi' three times daily. On day 19, under chloroform, the partially enucleated tumour was seized by vulsellum forceps, its intrauterine base incised by 2 inches and the capsule incised anteriorly. Blood loss was 'moderate'. On day 21 the ergot produced a 'powerful uterine action' for 5 h so that the woman refused further medicines. The effect was attributed to the mass having now been expelled from the capsule. By day 35, a large section of the tumour had passed through the cervix. By day 49 she had been pain-free for 2 days and the mass was in the vagina with attachment to the uterine fundus via a narrow pedicle. There was a copious discharge and great debility. Under ether, the mass was seized using vulsellum forceps and detached digitally. The uterine cavity was plugged with lint saturated with perchloride of iron. The mass measured 5 inches. The woman then made a rapid recovery.

Another surgical approach was to use cautery to create a slough of the uterine wall low on the cervix in order to release tension in the mass and relieve pain. One woman who had been receiving injections of ergot had such pain that rectal morphia was needed four times daily. 'Life could not under those conditions endure very long.' She begged that something might be done since life was unbearable. The tumour extended from the umbilicus to low in the pelvis, displacing the os backwards. Under chloroform, cautery was applied to the anterior aspect of the cervix until the substance of the tumour was penetrated. The patient was freer from pain than for a considerable time previously. After separation of the slough the soft uterine tissue was incised to enlarge the hole. The cautery was applied four times over a few weeks. Although the tumour remained 'as large as ever' the woman was greatly improved. 'Her general health is now fairly good, and she is able to earn her livelihood as a needlewoman'.

ABDOMINAL PROCEDURES

The development of the abdominal operation of oophorectomy had been introduced independently by Battey and Lawson Tait as a means of stopping menstruation and relieving gynaecological problems. It came to be known as Battey's operation and could be applied in some fibroid cases, but often the ovaries were inaccessible because of the tumour. Where it was possible, the effect was that of a surgical menopause with expected shrinkage of the fibroid. If the patient survived the procedure the results were good, but in 1883 the operation had a considerable mortality. In Lawson Tait's account of this operation he presented a series of consecutive case histories demonstrating major benefits for these seriously ill women[4]. The follow-up histories provided by the local physicians of the women included testimonies such as: she 'is now able to take short walks, and to go about a little among the poor of the parish. Before the operation she had not left her room for eleven years' and 'I consider her case a 'triumph of surgery'. Her pitiable condition and agonizing pain had excited the sympathy of all who knew her. She is now a quite transformed creature'. More dangerous was hysterotomy/hysterectomy which had then recently been used by Mr Spencer Wells and which was viewed by Dr Atthill as only to be tried *in extremis*.

In the 1900 publication entitled *A Short Practice of Gynaecology* by Dr Jellet of Dublin[5] we begin to see the emergence of the current procedures in their early forms, alongside the older methods. The medical approach was based on ergot in an attempt to stem haemorrhages but the effect was 'most uncertain and unsatisfactory in its action'. Operative measures could now be divided into palliative and radical. The three palliative measures were curettage, electrolysis and oophorectomy.

Curettage would remove the endometrium and possibly bring temporary relief. Electrolysis, introduced by Apostoli in 1886, involved placing an electrode shaped like a sound in the uterine cavity and another shaped as a pad on the abdominal wall. They were attached to a battery and a current of between 50 and 200 mA passed for 5 min twice a week. The treatment was reported to provide 'marked temporary benefit' but 'should be discontinued if not effective'[5]. The mechanism involved was thought to be either local chemical cautery, disintegration of morbid products or promotion of uterine contraction, thereby reducing blood flow to the tumour. Oophorectomy was now displaced by hysterectomy to remain a procedure only to be used where hysterectomy could not be used. 'It is coming to be recognized every day that a woman with a uterus and no ovaries suffers more after the operation both mentally, and physically, than a woman who has her ovaries and no uterus'.

The radical procedures were hysterectomy (ventral or vaginal) or myomectomy/enucleation. Ventral (abdominal) hysterectomy could be partial (subtotal) or total. It was not yet clear which of the abdominal hysterectomy methods should be standard practice but where a reasonable length of cervix was not available the total operation was favoured. Vaginal hysterectomy by itself was rarely possible, although Dr Doyen had developed a morcellation method which permitted mutilation of the uterus, thereby reducing its mass, and this was considered by some surgeons to be the operation of choice where the mass did not extend above the umbilicus.

Myomectomy/enucleation could be performed abdominally or vaginally, depending on the site of the tumour. The term enucleation remained in use for procedures where the uterus was incised and the myoma removed from its capsule, and myomectomy described the ligation of the stalk of a pedunculated fibroid. By 1900 they were being described as aspects of the one procedure and gradually the term 'myomectomy' dominated. Where a large fibroid was enucleated abdominally and the uterine cavity opened, it was advisable to suture the upper aspect of the uterus to the abdominal wall and to place a gauze pack in the large cavity and bring the gauze out through the lower end of the abdominal wound as a drain. With hysterectomy the greatest dangers were ureteric damage and haemorrhage. Haemostatis was an even greater problem with myomectomy and especially with enucleation, so the mortality was higher than with hysterectomy.

DEVELOPMENT OF CURRENT TECHNIQUES

The current surgical techniques of myomectomy and hysterectomy for fibroids are very much as evolved in the work of Victor Bonney and are well laid out by him in his monograph published in 1946[6]. In this book he paid tribute to the pioneering work of Dr Alexander of Liverpool who explored myomectomy techniques in the 1890s but whose work, which had a 9% mortality, did not attract followers. Bonney started performing myomectomy in 1913 when he removed six large fibroids at a Caesarean section. In 1923 he invented the myomectomy clamp to permit control of haemorrhage. By 1945 he had performed 806 operations with nine deaths (1.1% mortality) of which there were only two in his last 400 cases. His record was 225 fibroids removed from a single uterus[6]. Bonney's work on myomectomy had been so influential that by the 1940s Solomons and Solomons[7] stated that 'myomectomy is the operation advised in nearly all instances' and 'after the menopause, unless myomectomy is obviously a simple proposition, hysterectomy should be done'. The preferred method of myomectomy was Bonney's abdominal approach and although vaginal myomectomy had been further developed it was less favoured.

With hysterectomy there was still debate about whether the subtotal or total operation should be done. Subtotal hysterectomy had the advantages that the ureters were less endangered and a risk of infection from the vagina was avoided. The disadvantages were that the cervical stump could give rise to leucorrhoea and occasionally carcinoma. The prerequisites for the subtotal operation were nulliparity, a healthy cervix and no tumour in the cervix. The subtotal operation accounted for about 20% of the hysterectomies. As far as the ovaries were concerned it was felt important 'to be able to tell a patient she still has her ovaries. From the psychological aspect and possibly from the secretory aspect we deem it wise to leave them *in situ* when they are absolutely normal'.

In the 1944 account, in addition to the surgical approach, there was also the induction of a radiation menopause for women between 40 and 60 years old who were debilitated. Others favoured direct radiotherapy to the fibroids themselves. For palliation, ergot and curettage were still advocated.

By 1957 Dugald Baird[8] advocated palliation if the symptoms were mild, the tumours were small and if the woman was approaching the menopause, or the patient was debilitated. The range of options was: analgesia, iron therapy and blood transfusion. Testosterone had been reported to induce a temporary reduction in size. Radiation menopause continued to be an option but direct radiotherapy to the fibroids had been discarded.

By 1957 surgical methods were preferred, with the vaginal route used only for fibroid polypi. The abdominal options were myomectomy/enucleation where fertility was required, otherwise hysterectomy was favoured, particularly for the over 40s. Total hysterectomy was now standard 'unless there is a strong reason to the contrary', because of the risk of carcinoma developing in the stump. Since the blood loss at enucleation could be heavy, Baird advocated the use of Bonney's myomectomy clamp across the uterine vessels and ring forceps across the ovarian vessels. The clamps were released after full repair of the defects with interrupted sutures. Bonney's advice to remove as many fibroids as possible through a single incision placed in the anterior uterine wall had become standard teaching. This was to minimize subsequent adhesion formation. Before myomectomy Baird also advised curettage, to exclude fibroids involving the endometrium, and the testing of tubal patency which was retested 3 months later.

CONCLUSION

Bonney's work has remained influential to this day. We have had improvements in safety with developments in anaesthetic techniques, transfusion technology, perioperative drug options and suture materials but in many ways the operations have changed little for at least 30 and possibly 50 years. Today there would be general agreement that the only indication for myomectomy is the improvement in reproductive potential, otherwise total hysterectomy is the option if the fibroids are associated with menstrual disturbance, pain, bladder or bowel symptoms. The subtotal operation is now rarely used. Before myomectomy the woman must realize that there is a small risk that hysterectomy may be unavoidable. Before hysterectomy the fate of the ovaries must be considered and here there may still be scope for disagreement. I favour retention of healthy-looking ovaries in all premenopausal hysterectomies because the symptom consequences of the surgical menopause can be so severe. Most patients appear to agree with this approach. Whilst hormone replacement will alleviate menopausal symptoms, there are some women who have difficulty with it and, sadly, I have seem cases in whom hormone replacement was contraindicated and whose healthy ovaries were removed as routine practice. If ovaries are retained, oestrogen production is likely to continue and the risk of subsequent carcinoma is acceptably low.

I have shown that myomectomy and hysterectomy are part of a process of continuous development which will now include endoscopic resection and gonadotropin releasing hormone agonists. It is a tribute to Victor

Bonney that the practice was standardized for so long. I am sure both Sims and Bonney and the others of the past would welcome these new approaches, but we must maintain a critical stance to see if they are destined to stand alongside myomectomy and hysterectomy as standard techniques or eventually become historical sidelines along with vaginal enucleation and the radiation menopause.

REFERENCES

1. Monoghan, J.M. (1986). *Bonney's Gynaecological Surgery*. (London: Bailliere, Tindall)
2. Sims, J.M. (1866). *Clinical Notes on Uterine Surgery*. (London: Hardwicke)
3. Atthill, L. (1883). *Clinical Lectures on Diseases Peculiar to Women*. (Dublin: Fannin)
4. Tait, L. (1889). *Diseases of Women and Abdominal Surgery*. (Leicester: Richardson)
5. Jellett, H. (1900). *A Short Practice of Gynaecology*. (London: Churchill)
6. Bonney, V. (1946). *The Technical Minutiae of Extended Myomectomy and Ovarian Cystectomy*. (London: Cassell)
7. Solomons, B. and Solomons, E. (1944). *A Handbook of Gynaecology*. (London: Bailliere, Tindall and Cox)
8. Baird, D. (1957). *Combined Textbook of Obstetrics and Gynaecology*. (Edinburgh: Livingstone)

8

Endoscopic surgery

A. Gordon

INTRODUCTION

Uterine fibroids are found in 20% of women by the age of 40 and may lead to infertility, recurrent pregnancy loss, dysmenorrhoea and abnormal uterine bleeding especially if they are in a submucosal position. Valle[1] stressed the necessity for hysteroscopy in the diagnosis of submucous fibroids. He found them in 9.2% of all women whereas he had suspected them, on clinical grounds, in only 4.8%. Where women had abnormal uterine bleeding, the incidence was 16.2%.

The classical surgical management of intramural and partially submucous fibroids has been that of total hysterectomy if the woman has completed child-bearing, or abdominal myomectomy if she desired more children. This involved major surgery and a prolonged hospital stay and recovery period. Moreover, it produced a uterine scar which could then compromise the management of future pregnancies. Fibroids which were totally submucous and pedunculated could be removed blindly by polyp forceps or under direct vision by radially incising the cervix or performing vaginal hysterotomy after mobilizing the bladder.

SUBMUCOUS FIBROIDS

Hysteroscopy has been used as a diagnostic tool for several decades but in the past 20 years it has been used increasingly as a means of access to the uterine cavity for therapeutic intervention. Most early workers used scissors and forceps which were passed along an operating channel, or introduced freehand alongside the hysteroscope[2]. Norment and colleagues[3] suggested the use of a monopolar resecting loop for the removal of pedunculated submucous fibroids but did not describe any cases. Neuwirth[4] described a series of four cases using a modified urological resectoscope, while DeCherny and Polan[5] extended its use to the resection of sessile fibroids of less than 3 cm diameter.

Preoperative evaluation

Preoperative evaluation is essential. Hysteroscopy should be performed in all patients with abnormal bleeding in whom fibroids may be suspected. Endometrial biopsy is mandatory in the older woman; ultrasonography is necessary if the fibroids have a significant intramural component, and hysterosalpingography may be of help in assessing the size of the uterine cavity and its response to medical preoperative therapy. In deciding on treatment, the surgeon should take into account the number and size of the individual fibroids, their relationship to the uterine cavity, the percentage of the intramural component and the total area or volume of the uterine cavity.

Treatment strategy

If the fibroid is less than 2.5 cm diameter and less than 25% intramural, immediate resection or vaporization with the laser is straightforward. Small fibroids with a larger intramural component may be resected, with experience, as it is safe to remove up to a 0.6 mm depth of normal myometrium deep to the fibroid provided that the fibroid is not close to the cornua. It is easy to distinguish the difference in appearance between the fibroid and the surrounding myometrium, so complete removal can be assured.

If the fibroid is between 2.5 and 5.0 cm in diameter, or over 50% intramural, primary resection or ablation is neither easy nor safe. In these cases, preoperative treatment with gonadotropin releasing hormone agonists for 8 weeks should be given; the fibroid will then be smaller, less vascular and easier to remove. As resection proceeds, contractions of the uterine muscle cause the fibroid to be extruded from the uterine wall into the cavity and an increasing portion of it becomes visible. The resection or ablation may be continued until most of the fibroid has been removed but, frequently, it may become unsafe to remove all of the tumour. In this case the fibroid may be devitalized by drilling it with the Nd-YAG laser or with the electric knife, thereafter the patient should be treated with GnRH agonists for a further 8–12 weeks and hysteroscopy repeated. At the second operation, the fibroid is usually pedunculated, white and avascular and the removal or ablation can be completed easily and safely.

Results

Hysteroscopic myomectomy has been performed in 261 patients complaining of menorrhagia with an 87.7% cure rate[6–9]. In Corson's series, 24 out of 28 patients complaining of dysmenorrhoea were cured and infertility was cured in 41 out of 61 patients in other series[6,7,9,10].

Complications

The reported complications of hysteroscopic myomectomy are similar to the complications of endometrial resection or ablation. There may be fluid overload, dilutional hyponatraemia, uterine perforation with consequent damage to adjacent organs, haemorrhage or infection. A small number of cases of leiomyosarcoma have been reported. These were discovered on examination of the removed fibroid fragments – diagnosis which would have been missed if laser ablation had been performed.

SUBSEROUS AND INTRAMURAL FIBROIDS

Hysteroscopic surgery for submucous fibroids has been an accepted practice for over a decade. Laparoscopic surgery for subserosal fibroids has been practised for several years, but the indications to remove relatively small fibroids in that position are debatable. In recent years some laparoscopists have employed more aggressive surgery to remove intramural tumours up to 11 cm diameter, but the procedure has not yet become widely accepted.

Preoperative evaluation

Full clinical assessment is mandatory, with the indications for myomectomy being infertility and occasional pain or growth of the fibroid. A hysterosalpingogram should be performed to determine the status of the Fallopian tubes and hysteroscopy also to exclude the presence of co-existing submucous fibroids whilst ultrasonography will help to determine the number, size and location of the tumours. If the fibroids are not numerous, less than 11 cm diameter and not adjacent to the intramural segment of the tube, they may be suitable for laparoscopic myomectomy.

Treatment strategy

Preoperative GnRH agonists should be given to reduce the size of the fibroids, increase the possibility of conservative surgery and to diminish blood loss.

Subserous fibroids may be removed by coagulating the pedicle with bipolar or monopolar electricity and transecting it with scissors. The indications for removing such fibroids, especially if they are small, are debatable.

Intramural fibroids may be removed by incising the capsule with a monopolar hook or knife and then enucleating the fibroid by grasping it with forceps and peeling it out of its bed with forceps and scissor dissection. Bleeding points may be controlled with bipolar electrocoagulation. The cavity should then be closed, as in normal open myomectomy, by one or two layers of 3/0 vicryl sutures, tying the knots inside the abdomen with forceps or by the extracorporeal knotting technique of Semm. The wound may be treated with Tissucol to prevent adhesion formation, although this rarely occurs after laparoscopic surgery.

The fibroid should be removed from the abdomen either by enlarging the umbilical or suprapubic incision, by posterior colpotomy or by morcellation with a tissue punch. Alternatively, the fibroid may be pulled up against the abdominal wall with forceps and cut into several pieces with a scalpel inserted after enlarging the incision to allow removal through the wound or through an 11 mm diameter cannula.

McLucas[11] has described a combined laparoscopic and vaginal approach to posterior wall fibroids. The fibroid was prepared for myomectomy laparoscopically and the operation completed under direct vision through a colpotomy incision.

Results

Dubuisson[12] presented a series of 58 patients who underwent myomectomy between January 1990 and June 1991, 51 by laparoscopic surgery. The indications for surgery were the size of the tumour (35), infertility (19), bleeding (3) and co-existing endometriosis (1). Preoperative GnRH agonists were used in 31 cases.

He used sutures in 34 cases, and of the seven patients on whom he performed second-look laparoscopy, there were adhesions in only one. No patient had complications and the average hospital stay was 2.8 days.

CONCLUSIONS

The place of hysteroscopic myomectomy is well-established and there is now little place for abdominal surgery unless a submucous fibroid is over 5 cm diameter and situated deep in the myometrium. Laparoscopic surgery is not so well accepted, although with training in these new techniques and proper case selection, there appears to be no reason why tumours of up to 11 cm diameter (and which do not involve the intramural segment of the Fallopian tube) should not be removed in this way.

REFERENCES

1. Valle, R.F. (1983). Hysteroscopy for gynecologic diagnosis. *Clin. Obstet. Gynecol.*, **26**, 253–76
2. Neuwirth, R.S. and Amin, H.K. (1976). Excision of submucous fibroids with hysteroscopic control. *Am. J. Obstet. Gynecol.*, **126**, 95–9
3. Norment, W.B., Sikes, H., Berry, F. and Bird, I. (1957). Hysteroscopy. *The Surgical Clinics of North America*, **37**, 1377–86
4. Neuwirth, R.S. (1978). A new technique for and additional experience with hysteroscopic resection of submucous fibroids. *Am. J. Obstet. Gynecol.*, **131**, 91–4

5. DeCherny, A.H. and Polan, M.L. (1983). Hysteroscopic management of intrauterine lesions and intractable uterine bleeding. *Obstet. Gynecol.*, **61**, 392–7
6. Corson, S.L. and Brooks, P.G. (1991). Resectoscope myomectomy. *Fertil. Steril.*, **55**, 1041–4
7. Loffer, F.D. (1990). Removal of large symptomatic intrauterine growths by the hysteroscopic resectoscope. *Obstet. Gynecol.*, **76**, 836–40
8. Derman, S.G., Rehnstrom, J. and Neuwirth, R.S. (1991). The long-term effect of hysteroscopic treatment of menorrhagia and leiomyomas. *Obstet. Gynaecol.*, **77**, 591–4
9. Donnez, J., Gillerot, S., Bourgonjon, D., Clerckx, F. and Nisolle, M. (1990). Neodymium:YAG laser hysteroscopy in large submucous fibroids. *Fertil. Steril.*, **54**, 999–1003
10. Mencaglia, L. (1991). Myomectomy. Presented at the *II Biennial Meeting of the International Society for Gynecologic Endoscopy*, Barcelona, October
11. McLucas, B. (1991). Myomectomy via colposcopy with laparoscopic assistance. Presented at the *II Biennial Meeting of the International Society for Gynecologic Endoscopy*, Barcelona, October
12. Dubuisson, J.B. (1991). Laparoscopic myomectomy. Presented at the *Xe Journees Aquitaines de Perfectionnement en Reproduction Humaine*, Bordeaux, September

9

Neodymium–YAG laser hysteroscopic myomectomy

J. Donnez and M. Nisolle

INTRODUCTION

Laser energy has some advantages in the precision of tissue destruction that are not shared by the electrical energy used in resectoscopes[1,2]. The most popular laser in gynaecology has been the carbon dioxide (CO_2) laser, so it was natural that an effort was made to adapt this for hysteroscopic use. However, several features of the CO_2 laser make it impractical for this purpose. There are three reasons why the Neodymium-YAG (Nd-YAG) laser is readily adaptable for hysteroscopy myomectomy:

(1) The energy beam can be transmitted easily into the uterine cavity by means of a flexible quartz fibre;

(2) Laser energy can be transmitted to the tissue surface through a liquid distending medium; and

(3) Tissue may be penetrated to a controlled depth.

The depth to which tissue destruction will occur can be controlled by varying the power used[3,4] and this physical quality can be used for myomectomy and hysteroscopic myolysis[5,6]. The aim of this chapter is to describe the different techniques of hysteroscopic myomectomy.

MATERIALS AND METHODS

The quartz fibre used to carry the laser light is a 'bare' fibre. It consists of quartz surrounded by a thin plastic jacket, beyond which the tip of the fibre extends for several millimetres. The fibre is gas-sterilized or wiped with alcohol or cidex prior to use. The laser power is 80 W.

There are several hysteroscopic instruments for endometrial ablation. The disadvantage of the earlier ones used was their inability to remove debris by suction of the interior of the uterine cavity during the procedure. The presence of a deflecting arm is of limited value in allowing the fibre to be stabilized. New instruments are now available in which the telescope is inserted into two sheaths of different diameter – one for inflow and the other for outflow: this arrangement resembles the classic resectoscope[7] and permits the constant cleaning of the uterine cavity. This system has been called continuous flow hysteroscopy (CFH).

The technique the author uses to provide constant uterine distention involves attaching a plastic bag containing 3000 ml of 1.5% glycine solution to blood infusion tubing. The bag is then wrapped in a pressure infusion cuff, similar to that used to infuse blood under pressure. The tubing is connected to the hysteroscope. Since CFH has been used, no 'overload syndrome' has occurred and this very simple system, which does not require any sophisticated and expensive pumps, allows the surgeon to perform hysteroscopic surgery under good conditions. Following 8 weeks of therapy, hysteroscopic myomectomy is carried out with the help of the Nd-YAG laser. A Sharplan 2100 apparatus (Sharplan, Tel Aviv, Israel) is used for generating the laser beam with a power output of 80 W.

In total, 276 women aged between 23 and 40 years (mean 34 years) with symptomatic submucous uterine fibroids have been treated with a biodegradable gonadotropin releasing hormone (GnRH) analogue (Zoladex® implant; ICI, Cambridge, UK). The implants were injected subcutaneously at the end of the luteal phase in order to curtail the initial gonadotropin stimulation phase always associated with a rise in oestrogen. One implant was systematically injected at weeks 0, 4 and 8.

After the initial stimulation of oestradiol secretion, GnRH analogue administration resulted in a postmenopausal oestradiol concentration range of 15 ± 6 pg/ml. Throughout the treatment period, luteinizing hormone (LH) and follicle stimulating hormone (FSH) concentrations were significantly suppressed by 2 weeks of treatment. Recovery of ovarian secretion occurred, on average, approximately 10 weeks after the last injection[6].

RESULTS

Using the method previously described[6,8], the decrease of very large submucous fibroid areas was calculated. When more than one fibroid was present, only the largest was evaluated. In all cases except four, the fibroid area was decreased by an average 38%. However, the response was variable, ranging from 4 to 95%. These changes were significantly different ($p < 0.01$; decrease from the baseline area of $7.2 \pm 4.7\ cm^2$ to $4.4 \pm 3.5\ cm^2$ by 8 weeks of therapy). The mean fibroid area in patients with a pretreatment fibroid area $< 5\ cm^2$, with an area $> 5\ cm^2$ to $< 10\ cm^2$ and with an area $> 10\ cm^2$ decreased, respectively, from 2.6 ± 1.2 to $1.5 \pm 1.0\ cm^2$, from 7.0 ± 1.3 to $4.0 \pm 1.6\ cm^2$ and from 15.2 ± 7.5 to $9.1 \pm 6.1\ cm^2$. In all subgroups, a significant decrease ($p < 0.005$) was noted. There was no significant difference between the different subgroups.

Classification of myomas

According to hysterosalpingography data, submucosal fibroids were classified as:

(1) Submucosal fibroid of which the greatest diameter was inside the uterine cavity (Figure 1);

(2) Submucosal fibroid of which the largest portion was located in the uterine wall (Figure 2); and

(3) Multiple (> 2) submucosal fibroids; myofibromatous uterus with submucosal fibroids and intramural fibroids diagnosed by hysterography and echography (Figure 3).

Submucosal fibroid of which the greatest diameter was inside the uterine cavity
All patients ($n = 190$) underwent myomectomy by hysteroscopy and Nd-YAG laser. In all cases, except two, the operation was easily performed.

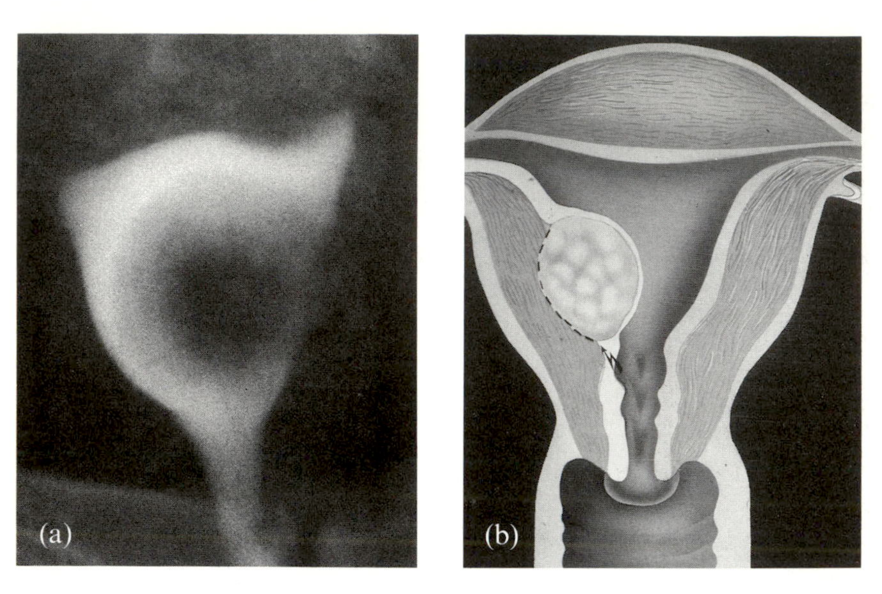

Figure 1 (a) Submucosal fibroid of which the greatest diameter is inside the uterine cavity; (b) Hysteroscopic myomectomy

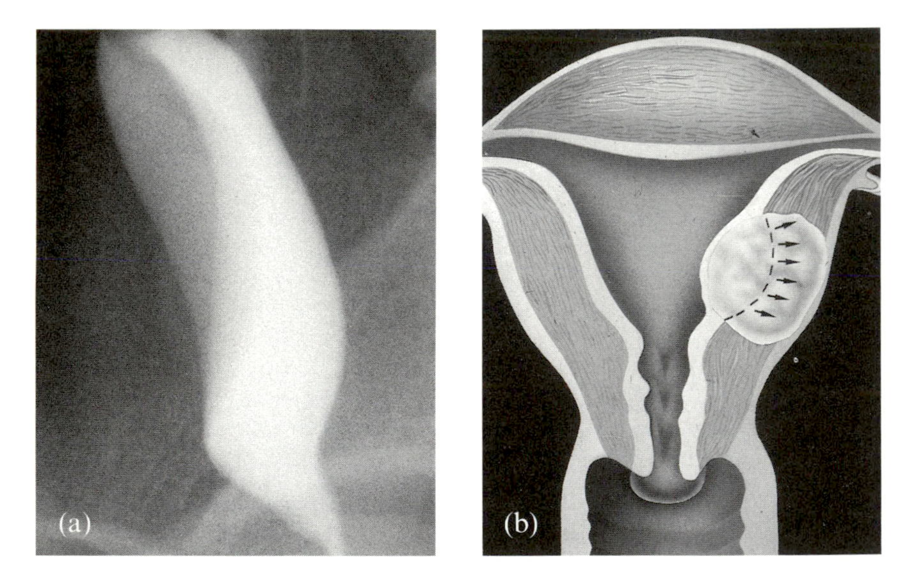

Figure 2 (a) Submucosal fibroid of which the largest portion was located in the uterine wall; (b) Hysteroscopic myomectomy: partial myomectomy and coagulation of the remaining intramural portion

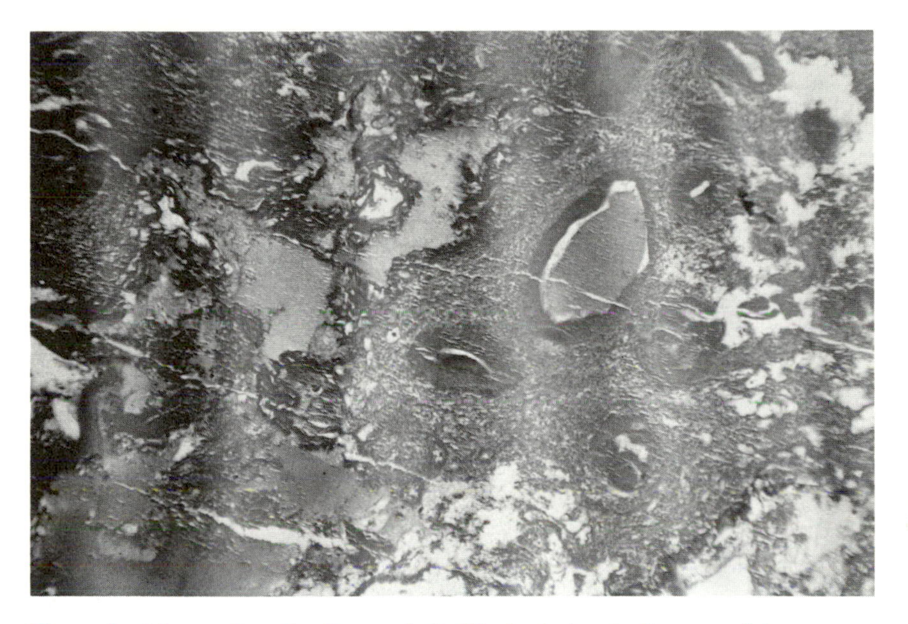

Figure 3 Myoma, 8 weeks after myolysis. Histological evaluation proved the presence of numerous areas of 'induced necrobiosis'

The myometrium overlying the myoma was less vascular and the 'shrinkage' of the uterine cavity may have accounted for the relative ease of separating the myomas from the surrounding myometrium (Figure 1).

The myoma was left in the uterine cavity. No complications such as infection, bleeding or uterine contractions occurred. Office hysteroscopy with the CO_2 laser, carried out 2–3 months after myomectomy confirmed the complete disappearance of the myoma, which was probably 'ejected' during the first menstruation occurring after the procedure.

No hormonal therapy, such as estrogens and progesterone, was given, and the operating time varied from 10 to 50 min (mean 24 ± 6 min).

Large submucosal fibroid of which the largest portion was located in the uterine wall

In cases of very large submucous fibroids in which the largest portion was not inside the uterine cavity but inside the uterine wall ($n = 54$) a *two-step operative hysteroscopy* was proposed[6]. After an 8-week preoperative GnRH therapy, a partial myomectomy was carried out by resecting the protruded portion of the myoma. Thereafter, the laser fibre was directed as perpendicularly as possible at the remaining (intramural) fibroid portion and was introduced into the fibroid at a length of 5–10 mm (Figure 2). During the application of laser energy, the fibre was removed slowly so that the deeper areas were coagulated. The end-point of fibroid coagulation with this technique was identified by distinct 'craters' with brown borders on all fibroid areas. The depth of the intramural fibroid portion was already well known due to echographic examination performed the day before surgery. The aim of this procedure was to decrease the size of the remaining myoma by decreasing the vascularity. This technique induces a myoma necrobiosis (Figure 3) and may be called 'transhysteroscopic myolysis'.

GnRH analogue therapy was given for another 8 weeks and the second-look hysteroscopy was then performed. In all cases, the myoma was again found to protrude inside the uterine cavity and appeared very white and without any apparent vessel on its surface. The shrinkage of the uterine cavity allowed the residual myoma portion to be easily separated from the surrounding myometrium and dissected off the myometrium. Myomectomy was then carried out and at the end of the procedure, the myoma was left in the uterine cavity. .

In all cases except five (< 10% of cases), the two-step therapy permitted the achievement of myomectomy. In the five exceptions, a 'third look' hysteroscopy was necessary to achieve myomectomy. When removed, myoma revealed areas of 'necrosis' on histological examination (Figure 3).

Fibromatous uterus

In cases of multiple submucous fibroids, each myoma was either separated from the surrounding myometrium or completely photocoagulated. When only a small portion of the myoma was visible, the fibre was introduced into the intramural portion to a length depending on the myoma diameter (diagnosed by echography). While firing, the fibre was slowly removed. Systematically, each myoma was destroyed. At the end of surgery, endometrial ablation with the Nd-YAG laser was carried out in order to induce concomitant uterine shrinkage. Endometrial ablation was carried out only in women > 35 years of age who did not wish to become pregnant subsequently.

When successfully performed, the myomectomy permits the restoration of normal flow. Long-term result evaluation shows that recurrence of menorrhagia was more frequent (22%) in cases of multiple submucosal myomas than in cases of unique submucosal myomas[9]. Recurrence of menorrhagia was provoked by the growth of myomas in other sites, as proved by hysterography and hysteroscopy.

DISCUSSION

In cases of submucosal uterine fibroids, hysteroscopic myomectomy is easily carried out if the greater diameter of leiomyoma, as assessed by hysterography, is inside the uterine cavity. A treatment duration of 8 weeks was adopted before hysteroscopic myomectomy. Indeed, in a previous study, a significant uterine shrinkage was observed at 8 weeks of therapy.

Because most leiomyomata return to near pretreatment size within 4 months after cessation of GnRH analogue therapy, these agents cannot be used as definitive medical therapy[10–13]. Several reports have demonstrated uterine and fibroid volume reductions of 52–77% after 6 months of GnRH analogue therapy, as assessed by ultrasound imaging. In our study, as documented by hysterography imaging, an average decrease of 35% in the uterine cavity area was found[8].

In cases of very large fibroids where the largest diameter was not inside the uterine cavity, the myomectomy was carried out in two steps. During the first surgical procedure, the protruding portion was removed and the intramural portion was devascularized by introducing the laser fibre to the myomas to a length of 5–10 mm, depending on the depth of the remaining intramural portion. The distance between the deepest portion of the myoma and the uterine serosa was evaluated by echography. The pelvic structures were protected from injury because the distance between the top of the fibre and the external surface of the uterus was never less than 1.5 cm.

A very interesting finding was that this intramural portion of the myoma became submucosal and protruded again inside the uterine cavity, possibly because of the GnRH analogue-induced uterine shrinkage, which provokes the protrusion of the remaining portion. In all cases, the largest diameter of the remaining portion was inside the uterine cavity so that myomectomy was easily performed by separating it from the surrounding myometrium using the Nd-YAG laser.

The peroperative blood loss was minimal, possibly because of decreased vascularity of the myometrium, which was demonstrated by a significant reduction in the uterine arterial blood flow (Doppler), after treatment with a GnRH analogue[14].

In conclusion, the use of GnRH analogues represents an adjunct for preoperative reduction of tumour size so that surgical treatment by hysteroscopy is possible. Even when the largest diameter is in the myometrium, the two-step hysteroscopic therapy combined with GnRH analogue therapy represents an ideal management of large submucous myomas and decrease the chance of myomectomy by laparotomy, which is often accompanied by operative blood loss and postoperative adhesion formation.

Other advantages in using a GnRH agonist preoperatively are, firstly, the restoration of a normal haemoglobin concentration and, secondly, the decreased risk of fluid overload[6,15].

REFERENCES

1. Hallez, J.P., Netter, A. and Cartier, R. (1987). Methodical intrauterine resection. *Am. J. Obstet. Gynecol.*, **156**, 1080
2. Loffer, F.D. (1988). Laser ablation of the endometrium. *Obstet. Gynecol. Clin. N. Am.*, **15**, 77
3. Goldrath, M.H., Fuller, T. and Segal, S. (1981). Laser photovaporization of endometrium for the treatment of menorrhagia. *Am. J. Obstet. Gynecol.*, **140**, 14
4. Goldrath, M.H. (1985). Hysteroscopic laser surgery. In Baggish, M.S. (ed.) *Basic and Advanced Laser Surgery in Gynecology*, p.357. (Norwalk: Appleton & Lange)
5. Donnez, J., Schrurs, B., Gillerot, S., Sadow, J. and Clerckx, F. (1989). Treatment of uterine fibroids with implants of gonadotropin-releasing hormone agonist: assessment by hysteroscopy. *Fertil. Steril.*, **51**, 947
6. Donnez, J., Gillerot, S., Bourgonjon, D., Clerckx, F. and Nisolle, M. (1990). Neodymium:YAG laser hysteroscopy in large submucous fibroids. *Fertil. Steril.*, **54**, 999
7. Neuwirth, R.S. (1983). Hysteroscopic management of symptomatic submucous fibroids. *Obstet. Gynecol.*, **62**, 509
8. Donnez, J., Schrurs, B., Clerckx, F. and Nisolle, M. (1989). Les agonistes de la LH-RH une alternative dans le traitement de la myomatose utérine. *Contracept. Fertil. Sex.*, **17**, 47
9. Donnez, J. (1992). Nd-YAG laser hysteroscopic myomectomy. In Diamond, M. and Sutton, C. (eds.) *Endoscopic Surgery*, in press

10. Healy, D.L., Fraser, H.M. and Lawson, S.L. (1984). Shrinkage of a uterine fibroid after subcutaneous infusion of a LH-RH agonist. *Br. Med. J.*, **209**, 267
11. Maheux, R., Guilloteau, C., Lemay, A., Bastide, A. and Fazekas, A.T.A. (1985). Luteinizing hormone-releasing hormone agonist and uterine leiomyoma: pilot study. *Am. J. Obstet. Gynecol.*, **152**, 1034
12. Andreyko, J.L., Blumenfeld, Z., Marschall, L.A., Monroe, S.E., Hricak, H. and Jaffe, R.B. (1988). Use of an agonistic analog of gonadotropin-releasing hormone (nafarelin) to treat leiomyomas: assessment by magnetic resonance imaging. *Am. J. Obstet. Gynecol.*, **158**, 903
13. Friedman, A.J., Barbieri, R.L., Doubilet, P.M., Fine, C. and Schiff, I. (1988). A randomized, double-blind trial of gonadotropin releasing-hormone agonist (leuprolide) with or without medroxyprogesterone acetate in the treatment of leiomyomata uteri. *Fertil. Steril.*, **49**, 404
14. Matta, W.H.M., Stabile, I., Shaw, R.S. and Campbell, S. (1988). Doppler assessment of uterine blood flow changes in patients with fibroids receiving the gonadotropin-releasing hormone agonist Buserelin. *Fertil. Steril.*, **49**, 1083
15. Van Boven, M., Singelyn, F., Donnez, J. and Gribomont, B.F. (1989). Dilutional hyponatremia associated with intrauterine endoscopic laser surgery. *Anesthesiology*, **3**, 71

10

Attempts at medical treatment of uterine fibroids

G. McSweeney and R.W. Shaw

INTRODUCTION

Because of the morbidity and mortality associated with the surgical management of uterine fibroids, attention has been directed towards the development of a safe and effective medical therapy. There are two main objectives in the medical treatment of uterine fibroids: relief of symptoms and reduction in fibroid size. The ideal end-point of medical treatment would be their complete regression but to date this has not been achieved.

Whichever medical therapy is used, and regardless of the degree of shrinkage, regrowth of the tumour occurs after discontinuation of treatment. Prolonged use of the various medical therapies used to date in the management of fibroids has been limited by side-effects. In certain women, medical therapy may be offered as a possible alternative to surgical intervention, i.e. for the symptomatic treatment of menorrhagia associated with fibroids in perimenopausal women, or for those women in whom surgery is contraindicated.

In most cases, however, medical therapy is utilized as an adjunct to surgery, with the aim of reducing surgical morbidity. A number of therapies have been shown to induce amenorrhoea (danazol and gestrinone), thus enabling women who are anaemic due to menorrhagia to increase their haemoglobin concentrations prior to surgery. Those agents that effectively reduce fibroid size make surgery technically easier and, in certain cases, may even allow the laparoscopic or hysteroscopic removal of fibroids, thus avoiding a laparotomy. In the case of a hysterectomy, preoperative shrinkage of fibroids may enable a vaginal, rather than abdominal, approach to be used.

Attempts to achieve a medical therapy for fibroids began in 1946 when Goodman[1] reported that administration of progesterone to seven women with uterine fibroids produced a decrease in the size of the tumour or of the uterus in each patient. Segaloff[2] in 1949, failed to confirm this phenomenon. In 1966 Goldzieher[3] demonstrated that growth of fibroids could be blocked and degeneration induced by using large doses of progestational steroids. More recently, Coutinho[4,5] observed a decrease in fibroid and uterine volume using the antiprogestin gestrinone. In 1983, De Cherney and colleagues[6] presented preliminary data, stating that danazol therapy resulted in shrinkage of fibroids. In spite of these attempts it was not until 1983 when Filicori and co-workers[7] reported on the use of gonadotropin releasing hormone (GnRH) analogues to shrink fibroids that medical treatment was widely researched. This paper aims to review the various medical therapies used for the treatment of uterine fibroids prior to the advent of GnRH analogues.

The therapies to be discussed include progestogens, androgenic steroids such as danazol and gestrinone, prostaglandin synthetase inhibitors and tamoxifen.

PROGESTOGENS

Clinicians have recognized for years that fibroids are dependent on oestrogen for maintaining their growth. In 1938, Lipschutz and co-workers[8] reported on the experimental induction of uterine and extra-genital subserous fibromyomas of the abdominal cavity by administration of oestrogens. In 1939, he announced that the development of this oestrogen-dependent tumour could be prevented, or the tumour made to disappear by the administration of progesterone[9].

Postulating that progesterone produced in the body may interact synergistically with oestrogen on the uterus, but also have antagonistic action, Lipschutz and his co-workers investigated the preventive action of several steroids on experimentally produced tumours[10]. Three different steroids – progesterone, deoxycorticosterone acetate and testosterone propionate were shown to have the capacity to prevent abdominal fibroids being elicited by oestrogens. The minimum quantity of steroid which has to be released to inhibit fibroid growth was lowest with progesterone. These results were in accord with clinical observations that fibroids are most frequent in nulliparous women. Their frequency was also reported to be greater in women who became pregnant at a more advanced age and had fewer pregnancies. It was assumed that the action of progesterone might exert a preventive influence in women with a greater number of pregnancies. In 1946, Goodman[1] reported seven cases of clinically diagnosed fibroids which regressed following therapy with injections of progesterone in doses varying from 10 mg three times weekly to 10 mg daily for periods of 2–6 weeks. However, this study was based on pelvic examination only and was poorly documented.

In 1942, Lipschutz again reported on the antitumourigenic activity of progesterone[10]. He and his co-workers had been studying the experimental tumour extensively and they emphasized several facts – notably that the tumour could be elicited by minute quantities of oestrogen, but that the action of oestrogen must be continuous rather then intermittent.

In 1949 Segaloff, in an attempt to evaluate progesterone therapy of human fibroids, treated six patients with progesterone for periods varying from 30 to 189 days. It was administered to three patients in the form of a daily intramuscular injection of 20 mg and to the remaining three by implantation of 200 mg of compressed pellets. This treatment did not affect the size of the uterine tumours, as demonstrated by contrast radiography. There was neither any microscopic evidence of increased involution in the fibroids removed at hysterectomy; in fact many showed considerable cellularity in their histological structure.

However, in 1966 Goldhiezer reported intense degenerative changes in myomata following large doses of progestogens[3]. He used medrogestone (25 mg) daily for 21 days in one group. This produced marked degenerative changes, but no mitoses or other signs of actual growth were seen. In a control group, which received 2 mg norethindrone daily for 30 days, no such changes were observed. No effort was made in this study to estimate the size of the fibroids before or after treatment and effectiveness was based only on histological findings.

Although it has been suggested that progestogen therapy may be efficacious in the treatment of uterine fibroids, this remains unproven at present. The number of cytoplasmic progesterone receptors in uterine fibroids has been reported to be lower than in normal myometrium[11].

This may explain why progesterone therapy has been relatively ineffective. Clinical studies are inconsistent and inconclusive, limited by the small numbers of patients and crude estimation of uterine and/or fibroid size.

Presently, the only role for progesterone therapy in the treatment of uterine leiomyomata may be in combination with GnRH analogue therapy following initial reduction in uterine volume by analogue alone. The addition of a progestogen to GnRH analogue therapy appears to decrease the incidence of hot flushes and to reduce the risk of osteoporosis in women requiring long-term analogue therapy[12].

GESTRINONE

Gestrinone is a synthetic trienic 19 norsteroid also known as R2323 which has been shown to be effective in the treatment of endometriosis. In 1981, Coutinho[4] reported a significant volume reduction of a pelvic leiomyoma and subsequent pregnancy in an 18-year-old infertile patient treated for 14 months with gestrinone (5 mg) orally every 2 days for 2 months, then twice a week for the rest of the treatment period. A more extensive study of 97 women was published by the same group in 1986. Group A patients ($n = 34$) received 5 mg of gestrinone twice a week whereas women in Group B ($n = 36$) received half that dosage at the same time. The remaining 27 women (Group C) received 2.5 mg vaginally three times weekly. The duration of therapy was variable. Some patients took the medication for 4 months, others for up to 13 months. Data on all patients were only available after 4 months of treatment with gestrinone. At that time uterine volume decreased by 18% in Group A and 27% in Group B but increased by 5% in Group C. Overall, the mean reduction in uterine volume was not impressive and fibroid volume was in fact increased or unchanged in 26 women. However, by the end of 4 months of treatment, 95 patients were amenorrhoeic and Coutinho recommended the use of gestrinone as a preoperative therapy to allow restoration of haemoglobin concentration by controlling excessive menstrual bleeding associated with fibroids.

DANAZOL

As treatment with danazol is effective in endometriosis with an oestrogen-dependent pathology, one might presume that it is useful in the management of uterine fibroids. At the 1983 Annual Meeting of the American Fertility Society, Professor Maheux presented the results of a study conducted at Yale University on the use of danazol in eight patients with uterine fibroids using 800 mg of danazol daily for 6 months. This substantial dose produced only a 20–25% reduction in uterine volume. They believed the poor results obtained might be explained by the fact that danazol has androgenic properties. Tamaya and colleagues[13], in 1979, demonstrated androgen receptors in uterine fibroids with an increased 5α-reductase activity when compared to the normal endometrium and myometrium. Yamamoto and co-workers[14] demonstrated, in 1984, that, unlike normal myometrium, fibroids have a high aromatase activity and are able to synthesize oestrogens from androgens. In fact Yuen[15], in 1981, reported the development of fibroids in a patient receiving 6 months treatment of danazol for endometriosis. These had been absent at the pretreatment laparoscopy.

TAMOXIFEN

In a study by Lumsden and colleagues[16], tamoxifen (20 mg per day) was administered to six premenopausal women with uterine fibroids for at least 3 months. Fibroid volume did not change significantly during treatment, being at 112.6% of their original volume after 3 months of treatment. Four subjects completed 6 months of therapy, after which fibroid volume was 115.5% of the original. However, menstrual bleeding was decreased subjectively in all but one subject.

ANTIPROSTAGLANDINS

Prostaglandin synthetase inhibitors reduce excessive menstrual bleeding in women with essential menorrhagia and menorrhagia associated with an intrauterine contraceptive device. Therefore, it is reasonable to assume that they may also be effective for myoma-induced menorrhagia. However, in a prospective placebo controlled study from Finland[17], Ylikorkala and colleagues showed the opposite; the utilization of naproxen (500–1000 mg daily) for 5 days had no effect of myoma-induced menorrhagia, although it reduced menstrual bleeding by 35.7% in women with idiopathic menorrhagia. This study was based on symptomatic assessment only, and fibroid size was not measured.

MISCELLANEOUS AGENTS

Gossypol

Meiling[18], in 1980, reported on the use of gossypol in 30 women with menopausal functional bleeding, uterine myomata or endometriosis. Oestrogen levels were lowered and in 70 cases endometrial sampling showed highly atrophied endometrium. In 62.5% there was a limited reduction of fibroid volume. However, the main concern with this agent is the possible side-effects. Fatigue and non-reversible hypokalaemia have been reported in clinical trials using gossypol for male contraception. A direct permanent effect of the gonad is also possible.

Amantadine

Amantadine is approved by the FDA for the treatment of Parkinson disease and drug-induced extrapyramidal reactions. It causes the release of endogenous dopamine and activates the dopaminergic and noradrenergic neurons. Luisi and Luisi[19] reported on their 10-year experience treating symptomatic fibroids with amantadine. A total of 160 patients received amantadine (200 mg daily) for 20 days a month for 6 months and these authors reported that after 6 months of therapy, the growth of the myoma was arrested, the consistency diminished and the symptomatology had subsided. The mechanism of action is unclear but it was considered that the reduction in tumour size was related to reduced blood flow. Although amantadine may be of value in the treatment of fibroids, its efficacy has not been demonstrated adequately and it does have known adverse reactions, including congestive heart failure, renal impairment and orthostatic hypotension.

CONCLUSION

Apart from GnRH analogue therapy, no other single medical agent appears to be of proven benefit in the treatment of uterine fibroids. The benefit of progestogens alone remains unproven, although their role in combination with GnRH analogues may be beneficial and is currently being investigated further. Tamoxifen may also prove to be of benefit in this context.

Danazol appears to have a very limited role in the management of fibroids apart from control of menorrhagia[20]. The same is true for gestrinone, which Coutinho recommended as a preoperative therapy, allowing patients to restore their normal haemoglobin concentrations.

Given the evidence from the literature, GnRH analogues appear to be the most effective agents currently available for medical treatment of uterine fibroids. With further research into the safety and efficacy of long-term GnRH analogue and hormone add-back regimes, it may well be possible to treat women with symptomatic fibroids.

REFERENCES

1. Goodman, A.L. (1946). Progesterone therapy in uterine fibroma. *J. Clin. Endocrinol. Metab.*, **6**, 402
2. Segaloff, A., Weed, J.C., Sternberg, W.H. and Parson, D. (1949). The progesterone therapy of human uterine leiomyomas. *J. Clin. Endocrinol. Metab.*, **9**, 1273
3. Goldhiezer, J.W., Maqueo, M., Ricaud, L., Aquilar, J.H. and Canales, E. (1966). Induction of degenerative changes in uterine myomas by high dose progestin therapy. *Am. J. Obstet. Gynecol.*, **96**, 1078
4. Coutinho, E.M. (1981). Conservative treatment of uterine leiomyoma with the anti-progesterone, R-2323. *Int. J. Gynecol. Obstet.*, **19**, 357
5. Coutinho, E.M., Boulanger, G.A. and Concalves, M.T. (1986). Regression of uterine leiomyomas after treatment with gestrinone, an anti-oestrogen, anti-progesterone. *Am. J. Obstet. Gynecol.*, **155**, 761–7
6. De Cherney, A.H., Maheux, R. and Polan, M.L. (1983). A medical treatment for myomata uteri. *Fertil. Steril.*, **39**, 429
7. Filicori, M., Hall, D.A., Loughlin, J.S., Rivier, J., Vale, W and Crowley, W.F. Jr (1983). A conservative approach to the management of uterine leiomyoma: Pituitary desensitization by a luteinizing hormone releasing

hormone analogue. *Am. J. Obstet. Gynecol.*, **147**, 726–7

8. Lipschutz, A. and Inglesias, R. (1938). Multiples tumeurs uterines et extragenitales provoquees par le benzoate d'oestradiol. *Compt. Rend. Soc. Biol.*, **129**, 519–24
9. Lipschutz, A., Murillo, R. and Vargas, L., Jr (1939). Antitumorigenic action of progesterone, *Lancet*, **2**, 420–1
10. Lipschutz, A., Vera, O. and Gonzales, S. (1942). The relation of the antifibromatogenic activity of certain steroids to their molecular structure and to various actions of these hormones. *Cancer Res.*, **2**, 204–9
11. Pollow, K., Geilfuss, J., Buquoi, E. and Pollow, B. (1978). Estrogen and progesterone binding proteins in normal human myometrium and leiomyoma tissue. *J. Clin. Chem. Clin. Biochem.*, **16**, 503
12. West, C.P., Lumsden, M.A. and Baird, D.T. (1989). LHRH analogues and fibroids – potential for longer term use. *Horm. Res.*, **32**, 146–9
13. Tamaya, T., Motoyama, T., Ohono, Y., Ide, N., Tsurusak, T. and Okada, H. (1979). Estradiol 17, progesterone, and 5-alpha dihydrotestosterone receptors of uterine myometrium and myoma in the human subject. *J. Steroid. Biochem.*, **10**, 615
14. Yamamoto, T., Takamori, K. and Okada, H. (1984). Estrogen biosynthesis in leiomyoma and myometrium of the uterus. *Horm. Metab. Res.*, **16**, 678–9
15. Yuen, B.H. (1981). Danazol and uterine leiomyomas. *Can. Med. J. Assoc.*, **124**, 963–4
16. Lumsden, M.A., West, C.P. and Baird, D.T. (1989). Tamoxifen prolongs luteal phase in premenopausal women but has no effect on the size of uterine fibroids. *Clin. Endocrinol.*, **31**, 335–43
17. Ylikorkala, O. and Pekonen, F. (1986). Naproxen reduces idiopathic but not fibromyoma-induced menorrhagia. *Obstet. Gynecol.*, **68**, 10–12
18. Meiling, H. (1980). Gossypol treatment for menopausal functional bleeding, myoma of the uterus and endometriosis: preliminary report. *Acta Adac. Med. Sin.*, **2**, 170
19. Luisi, M. and Luisi, S.V. (1982). Dystrophic effects induced by amantadine of uterine fibroleiomyomas. *Am. J. Obstet. Gynecol.*, **143**, 975
20. Oradell, N.J. (1987). *Physician's Desk Reference*, 41st edn., pp.1441. (Oradell, N.J.: Medical Economics Company)

11

GnRH analogues in the treatment of uterine fibroids: results of clinical studies

K.-W. Schweppe

INTRODUCTION

Hysterectomy is the most frequent major operation in gynaecology, and the uterine leiomyoma is the most frequent (> 30%) indication for this operation. In addition, uterine myomas may cause infertility, especially during the late reproductive years and may also complicate a pregnancy seriously. A review of nearly 2000 cases of myomectomy[1] demonstrated a 41% abortion rate prior to operation and a wide range of potential complications resulting from myomas in pregnancy, such as pain, haemorrhage, premature labour or rupture of membranes, and infection or degeneration of leiomyoma. The occurrence of any of these complications, especially repeated abortion, is an indication for the surgical removal of myomas. During recent decades, the classical approach in treating a young woman with symptomatic uterine myomas who wished to preserve her fertility was to perform a surgical myomectomy.

In some cases, this operation is easily performed – if the myomas are subserosal or pedunculated – but in most cases significant blood loss and postoperative formation of adhesions are common, especially if the leiomyomas are multiple or located deep in the myometrium. The pregnancy rate following classical myomectomy is only about 40%, and most babies are delivered by Caesarean section. The recurrence rate is as high as 15%, and secondary surgery is often needed.

Careful surgical techniques are necessary in order to reduce the risk of postoperative adhesions, and the injection of vasopressin around the myomas is recommended to avoid unnecessary blood loss. A new approach which minimizes blood loss is the preoperative use of gonadotropin releasing hormone (GnRH) analogues. Matta and colleagues[2] have shown a significant reduction of uterine arterial blood flow in women with uterine fibroids, as assessed by Doppler ultrasonography, following treatment with GnRH analogues.

Preoperative medical treatments

Since the success of myomectomy (in terms of pregnancy rate, full term delivery rate, low abortion rate and low recurrence rate) appears to be inversely related to the size and number of fibroids, it has been logical to assume that the preoperative shrinkage of tumours will result in a better prognosis. Therefore, preoperative treatment regimens with various drugs such as progestogens, danazol, gestrinone, etc. for ovarian suppression, have been reported. In general, the results have not been very impressive.

GnRH analogues: mode of action

The selective suppression of ovarian secretion of steroids by the repeated administration of gonadotropin releasing hormone analogues has been investigated as a new therapeutic approach in the medical treatment of uterine fibroids in recent years. Different degrees of successful regression have been reported in clinical trials[3–7]. The agonist can be administered intranasally or subcutaneously on a daily basis, or as a depot implantation every 28 days. Ovarian suppression may be variable and less effective when the drug is given intranasally[6]. From clinical evidence, the growth and regression of fibroids (i.e expansion during pregnancy, shrinkage after menopause) are oestrogen dependent; therefore a constant and effective ovarian suppression by subcutaneous application may result in a more effective regression of fibroids[5,6].

MATERIALS AND METHODS

This study describes the clinical results of a medical reduction of fibroids prior to surgery. In a prospective randomized trial, ten patients were treated with three doses of 300 μg buserelin intranasally every day and 12 patients received doses of 3.6 mg goserelin subcutaneously every 28 days for 3 months. To prevent hysterectomy, the indication was secondary infertility (13 cases) – repeated abortion may be caused by the fibroids, primary infertility (four cases) and hypermenorrhoea and dysmenorrhoea (five young women).

RESULTS

Ovarian suppression, as demonstrated by the reduction of the mean oestradiol level, was significantly more pronounced in the goserelin group 2 weeks after the initiation of therapy (Figure 1). Steroid production remained in the early follicular or menopausal range throughout the 3-month treatment period in all patients with means of 35 and 22 pg/ml oestradiol in the buserelin and goserelin groups respectively.

A variable response of the fibroids was seen in both groups; with buserelin we found four poor responders (Figure 2a) with a mean volume reduction of 18%, and with goserelin there were five poor responders with a mean shrinkage of 22% (Figure 2b). An effective reaction was achieved with buserelin in six women (Figure 3a) with a reduction of 48% (range 35–60%), and with goserelin in seven cases (Figure 3b) with a reduction of 64% (range 52–78%). The difference in the reduction of volume between the two treatments was statistically significant ($p < 0.01$). In all cases, an ultrasonographic examination after 4 weeks of treatment allowed the recognition of poor or good responders, because the relative percentage of shrinkage was highest at that point, and thereafter lower during the next 2 months of medication.

Hypo-oestrogenic side-effects (Figure 4) were reported more often in the goserelin group; general side-effects such as mood swings, headache and weight changes occurred at similar frequencies (< 20%) and were tolerable; only vaginal irregular bleedings were found with a cumulative frequency of 40% in the buserelin group and 10% in the goserelin group.

In the buserelin group, two patients had to be excluded from the study because of a violation of protocol; they refused the operation at the

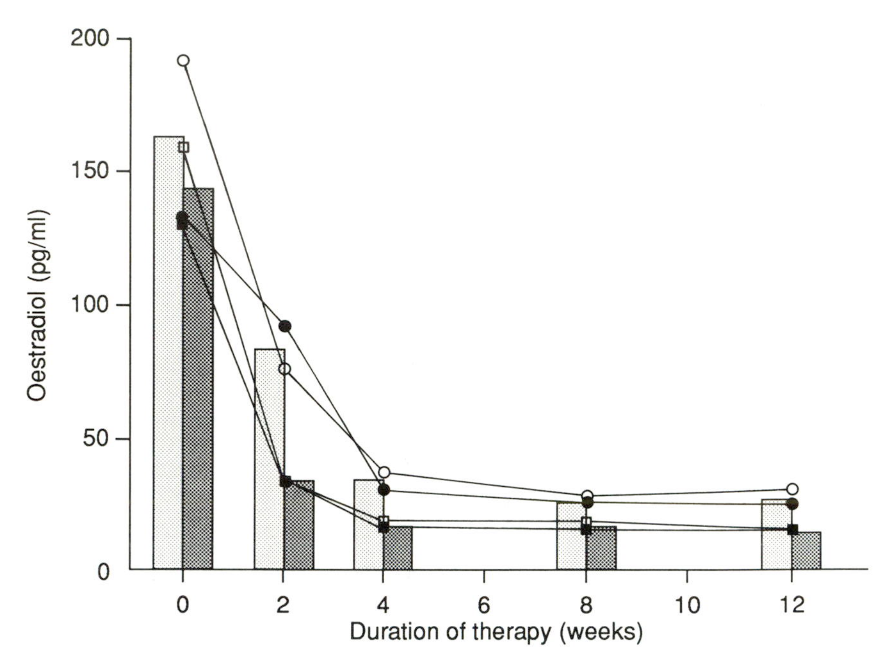

Figure 1 Ovarian suppression. Reduction of mean oestradiol levels in the buserelin-treated (light bars) and goserelin-treated (dark bars) groups. Individual data are shown for buserelin-treated patients 1–5 (●), 6–10 (○) and goserelin-treated patients 1–6 (■) and 7–12 (□)

completion of medical therapy. In parallel with the recurrence of ovarian steroid secretion, a regrowth of the myomas was observed in both cases (Figure 5), and with a delay of several weeks the patients agreed to the surgical procedure.

In the follow-up period of 1 year, 11 of the 17 women with infertility conceived (eight with secondary and two with primary fertility). To date, we have observed one first-trimester abortion, two cases with preterm labour (treated successfully, and culminating in deliveries after the 35th week of gestation), six pregnancies which ended with term deliveries, whilst two pregnancies are continuing.

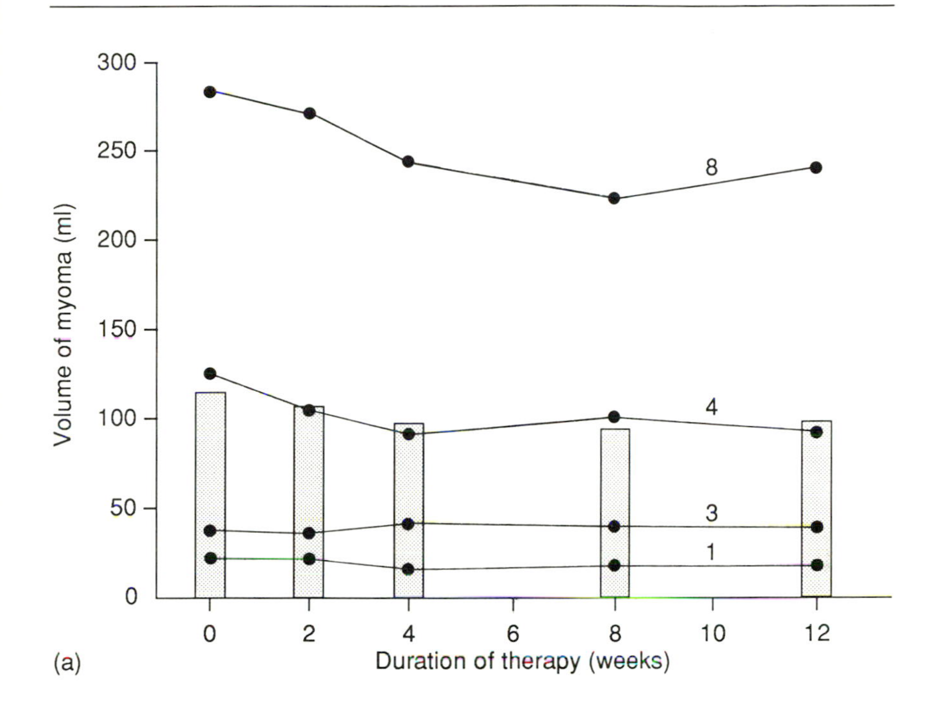

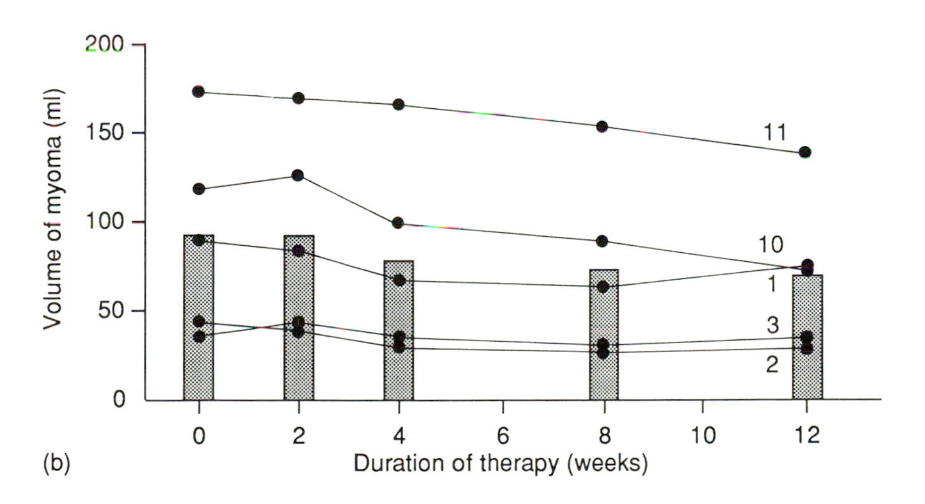

Figure 2 Myoma reduction in the buserelin-treated group (a) and goserelin-treated group (b): poor responders. Mean response is shown by bars and numbers indicate graphs for individual patients

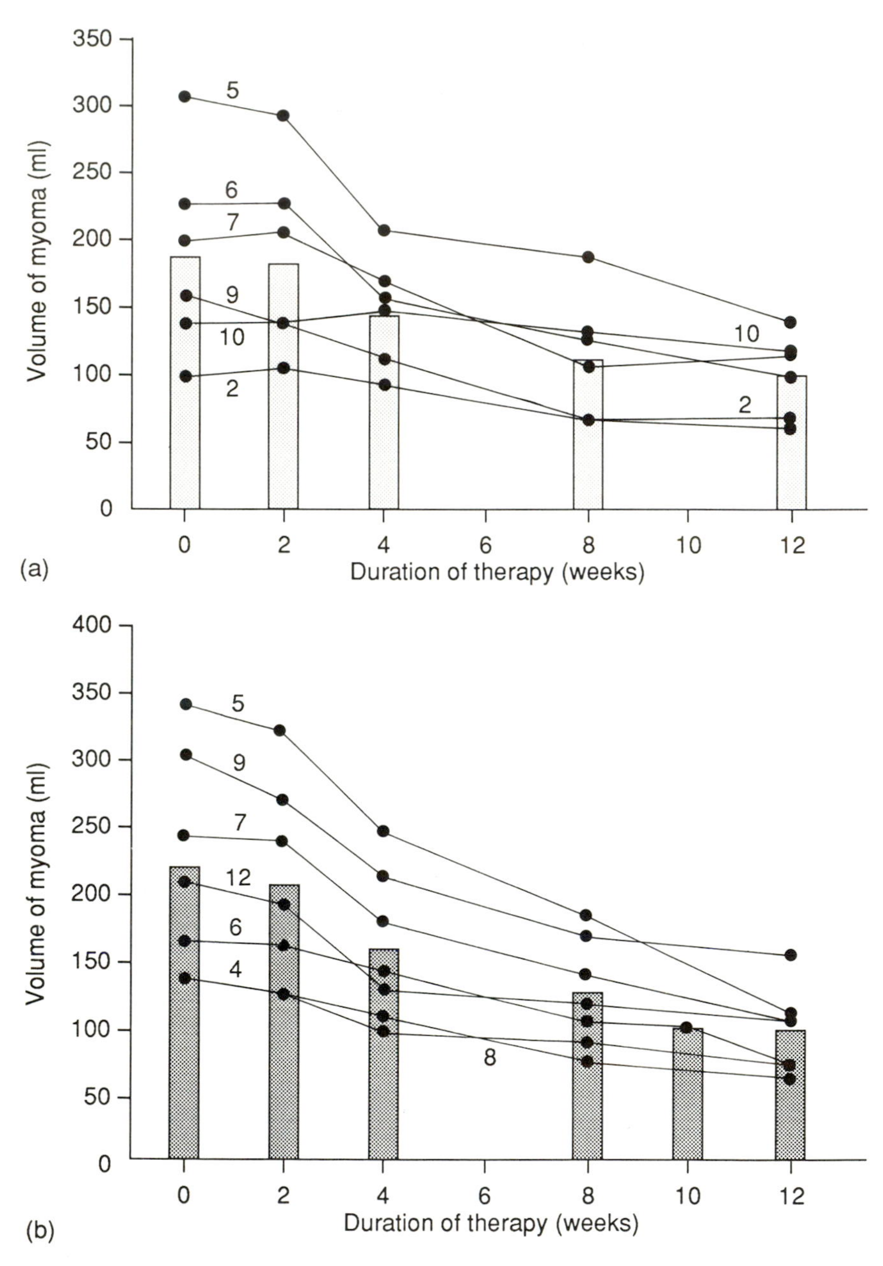

Figure 3 Myoma reduction in the buserelin-treated group (a) and goserelin-treated group (b): good responders. Mean response is shown by bars and numbers indicate graphs for individual patients

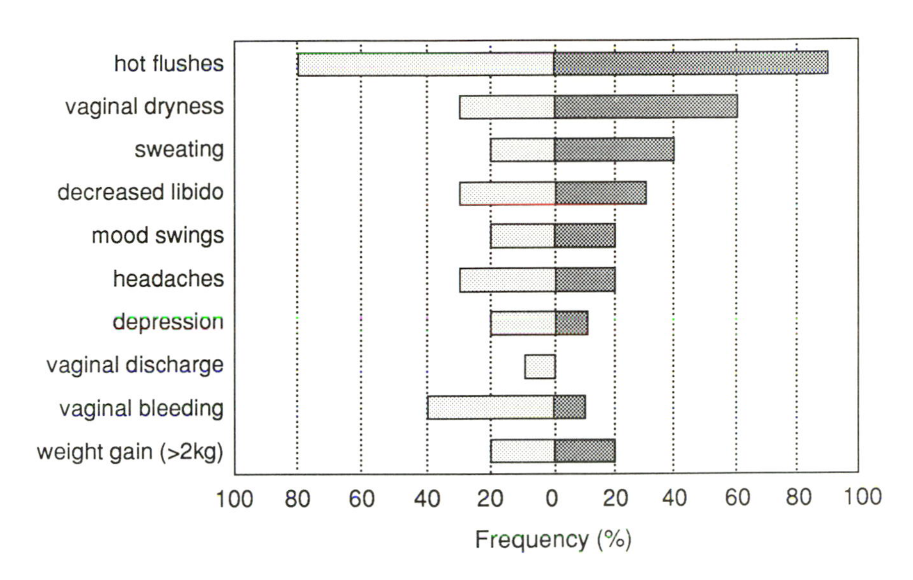

Figure 4 Side-effects reported by the buserelin-treated (light bars) and goserelin-treated (dark bars) patients

SUMMARY

The medical approach to preoperative treatment of uterine fibroids with GnRH agonists was effective in two-thirds of cases. Subcutaneous injection of a depot preparation, as compared with intranasal application, resulted in a more effective ovarian suppression and consequently in a more pronounced reduction of the volume of fibroids. Further studies must distinguish clearly between cases in which treatment for fibroids remains surgical, in which preoperative medical therapy is beneficial, and in which prolonged medication is indicated. Our present conclusion is that the shrinkage of fibroids caused by GnRH therapy is transitory only, and that rapid regrowth occurs in most cases. Therefore, we recommend this new therapeutic regimen for clinical use prior to conservative surgery only.

Currently under clinical investigation is the long-term treatment of fibroids with GnRH analogues as an alternative to operation (both myomectomy and hysterectomy). As demonstrated by Maheux[8], it makes little difference, with respect to the degree of fibroid volume reduction, if some basal oestrogen production by the ovaries is preserved. In terms of

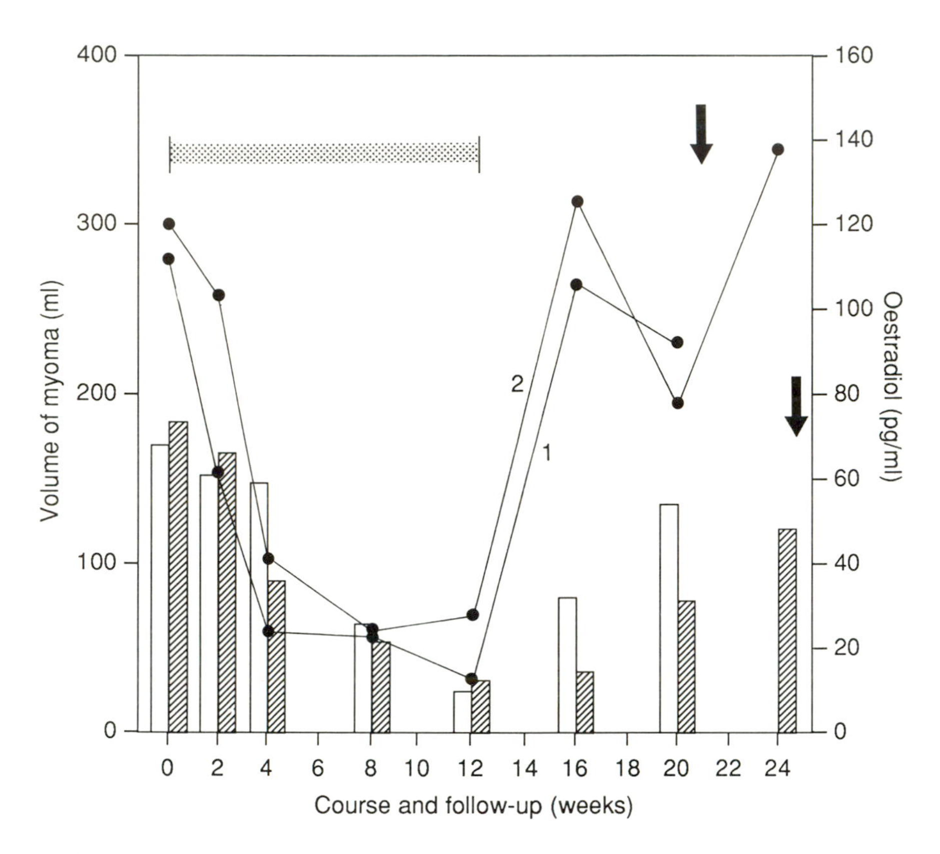

Figure 5 Regrowth of myomas and recurrence of oestradiol secretion in two patients (numbered graphs and patient 1 = clear bars, patient 2 = hatched bars) on completion of buserelin treatment (900 mg/day, shown by grey bar) and before surgery (arrows)

side-effects, however, he observed fewer hot flushes, increased high-density lipoprotein and no increased risk of bone loss. Therefore, new trials are underway to investigate a treatment combination of GnRH analogue with low-dose hormone replacement therapy after an initial 3-month ovarian suppression with 3.6 mg goserelin (monthly) alone. This approach may be an effective alternative to hysterectomy in premenopausal women with symptomatic uterine fibroids.

REFERENCES

1. Buttram, V.C. and Reiter, R.C. (1981). Uterine leiomyomata: etiology, symptomatology and management. *Fertil. Steril.*, **36**, 433
2. Matta, W.H.M., Stabile, I., Shaw, R.W. and Campbell, S. (1988). Doppler assessment of uterine blood flow changes in patients with fibroids receiving the gonadotropin-releasing hormone agonist buserelin. *Fertil. Steril.*, **49**, 1083
3. Maheux, R., Guilloteau, C., Lemay, A., Baeside, A.L. and Fazekas, A.T.A. (1984). Regression of leiomyomata uteri following hypo-estrogenism induced by repetitive luteinizing hormone-releasing hormone agonist treatment: preliminary report. *Fertil. Steril.*, **42**, 644
4. Henly, D.L., Lawson, S.R., Abbott, M., Baird, D.T. and Fraser, H.M. (1986). Towards removing uterine fibroids without surgery: subcutaneous infusion of a luteinizing hormone-releasing hormone agonist commencing in the luteal phase. *J. Clin. Endocrinol. Metab.*, **63**, 619
5. West, C.P., Lumsden, M.A., Lawson, S., Williamson, J. and Baird, D.T. (1987). Shrinkage of uterine fibroids during therapy with goserelin (Zoladex): a monthly subcutaneous depot. *Fertil. Steril.*, **48**, 45
6. Friedman, A.J., Barbieri, R.L., Benaceraf, B.R. and Schiff, I. (1987). Treatment of leiomyomata with intranasal or subcutaneous leuprolide, a gonadotropin-releasing hormone agonist. *Fertil. Steril.*, **48**, 560
7. Hackenberg, R., Gesenhuis, T., Deichert, U., Duda, V., Sturm, G. and Schulz, K.-D. (1990). Präoperative Reduktion von Uterusmyomen durch das GnRH-Analogon Goserelin (Zoladex). *Geburtsch. u. Frauenheilk.*, **50** 136
8. Maheux, R. (1989). Treatment of uterine leiomyomata: past, present and future. *Horm. Res.*, **32** (Suppl.), 125

12

Mechanism of action of GnRH agonists in the treatment of uterine fibroids

R.W. Shaw

INTRODUCTION

To date, the treatment of uterine fibroids has been primarily surgical as prior attempts at medical treatment have produced disappointing results (see Chapter 10). Myomectomy may be a complex surgical procedure because myomas are often multiple and those associated with symptoms of menorrhagia and infertility are likely to lie more deeply within the myometrium. The enlarged uterus may also be highly vascular, presenting problems of significant intraoperative blood loss. The formation of adhesions postoperatively may well then become a contributing factor to those patients seeking fertility – indeed fertility rates following myomectomy have been disappointing. In a review of 18 published studies of 1143 women undergoing myomectomy an overall pregnancy rate of approximately only 40% was achieved[1]. The authors of this review concluded that successful myomectomy seemed inversely related to the size of the myoma at the time of surgery and thus any treatment which may reduce fibroid size could well be beneficial to such operative procedures. Several studies have now shown the effectiveness of GnRH analogues in reducing the size of the leiomyomata[2–4]. Our own studies have confirmed these findings but we have also endeavoured to understand the mechanism(s) of fibroid size reduction during GnRH analogue therapy.

THE ROLE OF HYPO-OESTROGENISM

Little is known of the aetiology of uterine fibroids or the initiating factors stimulating formation and growth. It is presumed that their growth is dependent upon ovarian hormones, and in support of this hypothesis are their absence before the menarche, and their reduction in size following the menopause. Support for the theory that fibroids depend on oestrogen for continuing growth comes from a number of other sources. The relationship between chronic anovulation, endometrial hyperplasia, and the development of uterine fibroids has been reported[5]. Other studies have failed to demonstrate, however, any differences in circulating oestrogen, progesterone or gonadotropin hormone concentrations between women with fibroids and healthy controls[6]. Histological studies have demonstrated that hyperplastic changes are commonly present at the margins of fibroids where they co-exist in areas of normal and/or atrophic endometrium[7]. Thus, changes may reflect local differences in the binding of steroids in fibroid tissue and, indeed, higher concentrations of oestrogen receptors have been reported in fibroid tissue compared with adjacent myometrium[8]. Therefore the state of reduced oestrogen secretion may result in reduction in the growth of fibroids and induce regression similar to that observed after the menopause. We have performed a number of studies utilizing the GnRH analogues: D-Ser(tBu^6) Pro^9 NET LHRH (buserelin); D-(Nal$_2$)^6 LHRH (nafarelin); D-Ser(tBu^6)-Aza Gly LHRH (goserelin)[9–11]. In all of these studies, comparable degrees of reduction in uterine fibroid volume have been induced but with quite differing degrees of suppression of circulating 17β-oestradiol.

The administration of a monthly depot of goserelin (3.6 mg) induces a greater suppression of circulating oestradiol than buserelin or nafarelin administered intranasally. Despite this greater suppression of circulating 17β-oestradiol there appears no greater reduction in fibroid size when hypo-oestrogenism is more profound. Furthermore, the reduction in uterine size would seem to be maximal during the first month of treatment with GnRH analogues (Figure 1). This is more remarkable since the first 10–14 days following exposure to a GnRH analogue during the 'agonistic phase' is a period of increased levels of oestradiol within the circulation. Even at the end of 1 month's administration when down-regulation of the pituitary has been achieved, suppression of circulating 17β-oestradiol is still not maximal, and this may not occur until the

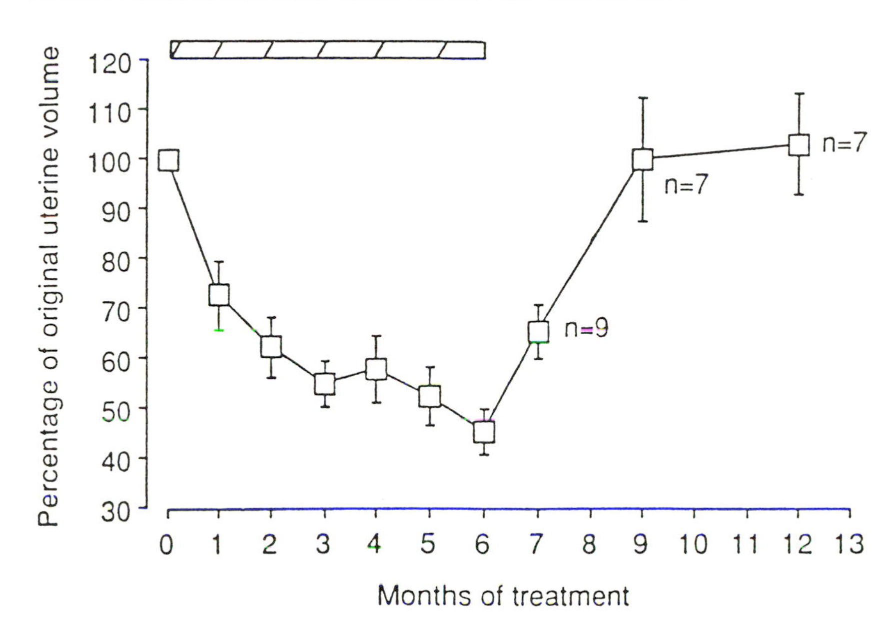

Figure 1 Mean reduction of uterine volume in 13 patients treated for 6 months (hatched bar) with intranasal nafarelin (200 μg twice a day) and subsequent changes during follow-up after treatment. (Reproduced from ref. 10, with permission)

second or third month of administration. The monthly percentage reduction in uterine fibroid volume in patients treated with the analogue nafarelin is shown in Table 1. By the third and fourth month of administration, maximum reduction in size has been achieved with no significant reduction occurring with further treatment in the majority of patients.

Following discontinuation of GnRH analogue therapy, oestradiol levels soon return to pretreatment levels with the return of ovarian function. Between 4–8 weeks after discontinuation of therapy, oestradiol levels are back to normal pretreatment follicular phase values. With the return of ovarian function, there is also a noted rapid regrowth, such that within 3 months of discontinuing treatment, fibroids return to their pretreatment size in the majority of patients.

Thus, induction of hypo-oestrogenism appears to be an important factor in inducing regression of fibroids, and an increase in oestradiol a factor in their regrowth. The effects of acute changes in oestradiol on uterine volume are apparent in Figure 2 in the case of one patient who

Table 1 Monthly reduction in uterine volume in patients with fibroids receiving nafarelin: 200 μg twice a day, intranasally ($n = 13$)

Month	*Mean (± SD) reduction* (%)
First	26.5 ± 10.1
Second	10.2 ± 6.5
Third	3.8 ± 4.1
Fourth	0.9 ± 1.2

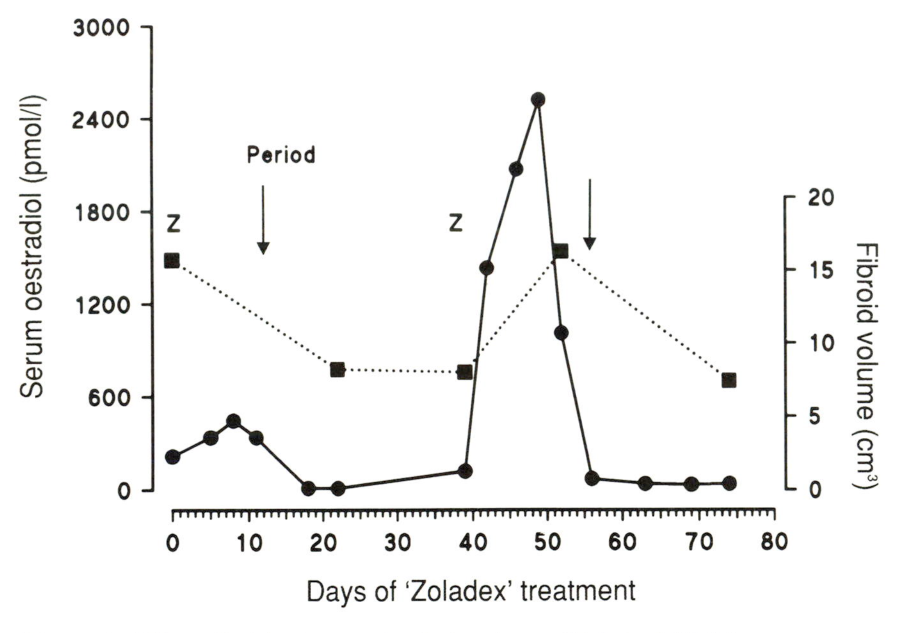

Figure 2 Effects of a delay in receiving further depot of Zoladex® (Z) 3.6 mg at correct time. Second depot induced agonistic rise in serum oestradiol (●—●) and rapid regrowth of fibroid (■······■), with further reductions when down-regulation re-established

commenced suppression with the depot analogue Zoladex®, inducing an initial reduction in fibroid size, then failed to return for the second depot to be placed. Subsequent administration of the depot, at a time when the pituitary was returning to normal function following desensitization, produced an exaggerated agonist response with increased oestrogen in the circulation following administration of the second depot. This induced a rapid regrowth of the fibroid over a period of 10–14 days, and subsequent shrinkage following the attainment of desensitization.

Reduction in total uterine volume or fibroid volume is dependent upon the lowering of circulating 17β-oestradiol levels. Patients failing to achieve adequate down-regulation with GnRH analogue therapy fail to demonstrate maximal reduction in uterine size. However, further reduction below a 'threshold level' of hypo-oestrogenaemia needed to gain a response does not induce a greater reduction in myoma size. Indeed, approximately 10% of fibroids fail to demonstrate significant reduction and this lack of response can be predicted by the end of the first month of treatment with GnRH analogues.

Recent evidence from women who have been rendered hypo-oestrogenic with GnRH agonists suggests that the oestrogen effect within fibroids is not direct, but rather is mediated via growth factors such as epidermal growth factor (EGF)[12]. This factor is known to control cellular proliferation implicated in tumour growth; high affinity binding sites for EGF are present in the uterus and oestrogen has been shown to influence this binding to fibroids but not to normal myometrium[13]. One report has also demonstrated specific binding sites for GnRH within fibroids[14], but these sites need to be confirmed by other studies before it can be assumed that there may be a direct action of GnRH analogues within fibroids.

DOPPLER ASSESSMENT OF UTERINE ARTERY BLOOD FLOW CHANGES

The rapidity of change in uterine volume (both of reduction and regrowth) suggests that factors other than cellular atrophy or hyperplasia play a part. It is possible that the reduction in uterine volume is partly related to induced changes in uterine blood flow. We studied the uterine arterial blood-flow velocity waveforms with Doppler ultrasound in patients with large uterine fibroids[15]. Eight patients presenting with 16–18 weeks pregnancy-size fibroid uteri were commenced on 400 μg of buserelin, intranasally, 8-hourly for a period of 4 months. Clinical estimates of uterine size, together with ultrasound uterine volume measurements, and of serum oestradiol, were measured before treatment, at 2 and 4 months of treatment, and 6 weeks after treatment. Doppler assessment of the impedance of blood flow within the uterine vasculature was carried out before treatment, and at monthly intervals throughout treatment. Photographs of the waveforms obtained at peak systole (A) and peak diastole (B) were measured to calculate the resistance index (RI = A–B/A), which reflects vascular resistance. These measurements were performed by a single observer taking the mean of three measurements each time with a coefficient of variance of between 3 and 5%.

Doppler ultrasound is an established technique in evaluating the impedance to flow (as measured by the resistance index) which has an inverse relationship to blood flow[16]. These results demonstrated that a reduction of total uterine and individual fibroid volumes in patients receiving GnRH analogues was associated with a corresponding increase in impedance to flow in the uterine arterial vasculature (Table 2).

Animal studies on the physiological effect of oestrogen on uterine vascular response have firmly established that the addition of oestrogen can directly cause vasodilation and increased blood flow in uterine vessels[17]. Our data from these Doppler ultrasound studies confirm that a reduction in circulating oestrogen levels leads to the opposite effect – that of vasoconstriction with reduced flow in the uterine vasculature. This might suggest that a reduction in the size of uterine fibroids, whilst associated with hypo-oestrogenism, may in part be related to reduced blood supply and vascular pools within fibroids. In addition, reduced blood flow to the fibroids may induce the hypoplasia of the smooth muscle components observed in many such treated fibroids (see below) and is certainly a contributing factor in the reduced measured blood loss during surgical removal (myomectomy) (see Chapter 13).

HISTOLOGICAL EXAMINATION OF FIBROIDS EXPOSED TO GnRH ANALOGUE THERAPY

Fibroids consist of varying proportions of smooth muscle fibres, collagenous/fibrous tissue components, vascular pools and areas of

Table 2 Changes in Doppler waveform velocity observed during treatment with buserelin: 400 μg 3 times a day, intranasally ($n = 8$). Figures are means ± SD

	Pretreatment	*2 months*	*4 months*	*2 months post-treatment*
Serum oestradiol-17β (pmol/l)	302 ± 43	116 ± 24	82 ± 23	297 ± 36
Total uterine volume (cm^3)	656 ± 113	487 ± 98	386 ± 70	501 ± 124
Mean (and SD) uterine arterial resistance index (RI)	0.52 (0.02)	0.68 (0.04)	0.92 (0.04)	0.59 (0.03)

calcification and degeneration. It had been hoped that a detailed study of these various components might give an insight into the mode of action of GnRH analogues. This has been discussed in Chapter 3, and it is apparent that there is great heterogeneity of histological features both within and between individuals, which makes specific interpretation of these changes difficult.

In many patients treated with a GnRH analogue for 3 months prior to myomectomy, light microscopy shows an alteration in the proportion of smooth muscle to fibrous components within the fibroids, with the nuclei of the smooth muscle fibres becoming more apparent and crowded in these patients compared with controls, simply because of a reduction in the cytoplasmic component of the smooth muscle fibres. This is more obvious in some patients when evaluated by electron microscopy where the majority of smooth muscle cells consists of the nuclei, which otherwise appear normal, and only a small surrounding area of cytoplasm (Figure 3). The general features are those of hypoplasia of these smooth muscle cells and no reduction in the number of smooth muscle cells or evidence of degeneration or necrosis within them. A detailed analysis of the vascular components show that increased areas of degeneration and necrosis are extremely variable in different patients, and even within patients whose fibroids have shown comparable degrees of reduction in size during GnRH analogue pretreatment. These histological and electron microscopy studies

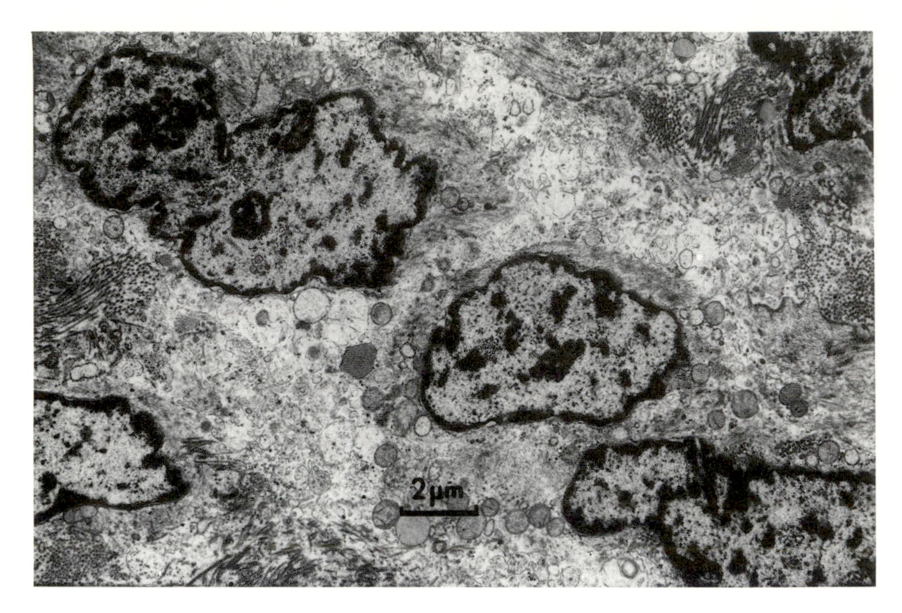

Figure 3 Electron photomicrograph of smooth muscle fibres within a fibroid removed following 4 months of pretreatment with Zoladex® (3.6 mg depot monthly)

to date, therefore, give no consistent insight into the mechanism of action of GnRH analogues in inducing this shrinkage.

CONCLUSION

In the majority of instances, treatment of uterine fibroids with GnRH analogues will result in a reduction of total uterine volume and individual fibroid volume. However, on discontinuation of analogue therapy, uterine size and fibroid regrowth return to pretreatment levels within a relatively short period of time.

It would appear that hypo-oestrogenism induced by GnRH analogues leads to a reduction of uterine arterial blood flow, and this may contribute to the reduction in size by reducing the vascular component within the fibroids, the reduced vascularity perhaps also being a factor in the hypoplasia of the smooth muscle component. A better understanding of the role of various growth factors is essential for us to try further to determine the mechanism of action of GnRH analogues in inducing regression of uterine fibroids.

REFERENCES

1. Buttram, V.C. and Reiter, R.C. (1981). Uterine leiomyomata: etiology, symptomatology and management. *Fertil. Steril.*, **36**, 433–45
2. Filicori, M., Hall, D.A., Loughlin, J.S., Rivier, J., Vale, W. and Crowley, W.F. Jr. (1983). A conservative approach to the management of uterine leiomyoma: pituitary desensitization by a luteinizing hormone-releasing hormone analogue. *Am. J. Obstet. Gynecol.*, **147**, 726–7
3. Maheux, R., Guillotea, C., Lemay, A., Bastide, A. and Fazekas, A.T.A. (1985). Luteinizing hormone-releasing hormone agonist and uterine leiomyomata: a pilot study. *Am. J. Obstet. Gynecol.*, **152**, 1034–8
4. Healy, D.L., Lawson, S.R., Abbott, M., Baird, D.T. and Fraser, H.M. (1986). Toward removing uterine fibroids without surgery: subcutaneous infusion of a luteinizing hormone-releasing hormone agonist commencing in the luteal phase. *J. Clin. Endocrinol. Metab.*, **63**, 619–25
5. Withersoon, J.T. (1935). The hormonal origin of uterine fibroids: an hypothesis. *Am. J. Cancer*, **24**, 402–6
6. Maheux, R., Lemay-Turcot, L. and Lemay, A. (1986). Daily follicle-stimulating hormone, luteinizing hormone, estradiol, and progesterone in ten women harbouring uterine leiomyomas. *Fertil. Steril.*, **46**, 205–8
7. Farrer-Brown, G., Belby, J.O.W. and Tarbit, M.H. (1971). Venous changes in the endometrium of myomatous uteri. *Obstet. Gynecol.*, **38**, 743–51
8. Wilson, E.A., Yang, F. and Rees, E.D. (1980). Estradiol and progesterone binding in uterine leiomyomata and in normal uterine tissue. *Obstet. Gynecol.*, **55**, 20–4
9. Matta, W.H.M., Shaw, R.W. and Nye, M. (1989). Long-term follow-up of patients with uterine fibroids after treatment with the LHRH agonist buserelin. *Br. J. Obstet. Gynaecol.*, **96**, 200–6
10. Williams, I.A. and Shaw, R.W. (1990). Effect of Nafarelin on uterine fibroids measured by ultrasound and magnetic resonance imaging. *Eur. J. Obstet. Gynaecol. Reprod. Biol.*, **34**, 111–17
11. Shaw, R.W. (1989). Mechanism of LHRH Analogue Action in Uterine Fibroids. *Horm. Res.*, **32** (Suppl. 1), 150–3
12. Lumsden, M.A., West, C.P., Bramley, T.A., Rumgay, L. and Baird, D.T. (1988). The binding of epidermal growth factor to the human uterus and leiomyomata in women rendered hypo-oestrogenic by continuous administration of an LHRH agonist. *Br. J. Obstet. Gynaecol.*, **95**, 299–304
13. Lumsden, M.A., West, C.P., Hawkins, T.A., Bramley, T.A., Rumgay, L. and Baird, D.T. (1989). The binding of steroids to myometrium and leiomyomata (fibroids) in women treated with gonadotrophin-releasing

hormone agonist Zoladex (ICI 118640). *J. Endocrinol.*, **121**, 389–96

14. Wiznitzer, A., Marback, M., Hazum, B., Insler, V., Sharoni, Y. and Levy, J. (1988). Gonadotropin releasing hormone specific binding sites in uterine leiomyomata. *Biochem. Biophys. Res. Comm.*, **152**, 1326–31
15. Matta, W.H.M., Stabile, I., Shaw, R.W. and Campbell, S. (1988). Doppler assessment of uterine blood flow changes in patients with fibroids receiving the gonadotrophin-releasing hormone agonist buserelin. *Fertil. Steril.*, **49**, 1083–5
16. Griffin, D., Cohen-Overbeek, T. and Campbell, S. (1983). Fetal utero-placental blood flow. *Clin. Obstet. Gynecol.*, **10**, 565–74
17. Resnik, R., Killam, A.P., Battaglia, F.C., Makowski, E.L. and Meschia, G. (1974). The stimulation of uterine blood flow by various estrogens. *Endocrinology*, **94**, 1192–7

13

GnRH agonists and blood loss at surgery

R.L. Gardner and R.W. Shaw

INTRODUCTION

Fibroids are the commonest tumour in the human body, and consequently symptoms attributable to such a common pathology – namely menorrhagia, pelvic–abdominal masses, pressure symptoms on the bowel and bladder and possibly infertility – present a major work load in the gynaecological outpatient departments. Uterine fibroids are the commonest abnormality given as a reason for hysterectomy. The surgical approach to treating uterine fibroids consists of hysterectomy and myomectomy. More recently, laser ablation of fibroids and hysteroscopic and laparoscopic myomectomy have been used to treat suitably sized and sited fibroids.

Both hysterectomy and myomectomy have a significant morbidity associated with the procedures. Myomectomy in particular has a high risk of intra-operative and postoperative haemorrhage associated with it. This may lead to hysterectomy, which is undesirable since myomectomy would have been chosen originally to retain the uterus, either because the patient had declined hysterectomy or because she wished to retain her fertility. Adhesion formation commonly occurs as a result of continued oozing from the uterine incisions in the immediate postoperative period. This may, in turn, lead to chronic abdominal pain and bowel symptoms and to tubal damage, lessening still further the chance of a spontaneous pregnancy. Methods have therefore been sought to make surgical procedures for myomectomy safer and to lessen the morbidity associated with such procedures.

GnRH AGONISTS AND FIBROIDS

Gonadotropin releasing hormone (GnRH) agonists have been known to shrink fibroids through their action which produces a state of hypogonadotropic-hypogonadism[1]. Their prolonged use desensitizes the pituitary, reducing follicle stimulating hormone (FSH) and luteinizing hormone (LH) levels, and thereby reducing the level of oestrogen[2]. This, in turn, has been shown by Matta and colleagues to reduce uterine artery blood flow[3]. Fibroids are known to reduce in size after the menopause for many years and the use of the GnRH agonists to produce a reversible menopausal state have recently been investigated widely, as a means of shrinking fibroids. After stopping treatment with GnRH agonists, however, the levels of FSH, LH and oestradiol return to normal, the fibroids regrow and may exceed their previous volumes rapidly, and the symptoms observed previously by the individual return[4]. The duration of such a course of treatment is limited by the bone loss associated with the prolonged use of a GnRH agonist[5,6], thus making the treatment unsuitable for long-term use as a conservative method of treating fibroids. The GnRH agonists may be of use in relieving symptoms in the short term, whilst the patient awaits surgery, or if the menopause is imminent.

GnRH AGONISTS AND THEIR INFLUENCE ON BLOOD LOSS AT SURGERY

Since fibroids shrink with the use of GnRH agonists, it would seem logical to investigate the beneficial effect of shrinking fibroids and to make use of the decreased uterine artery blood flow in patients undergoing hysterectomy or myomectomy, since it seems likely that this effect of the GnRH agonists may reduce blood loss at operation, thereby reducing the incidence of blood transfusion and perioperative morbidity.

At the Royal Free Hospital in London, 42 premenopausal women with fibroids (confirmed with ultrasound scanning) were recruited for a study of the influence of the depot GnRH agonist goserelin (Zoladex® depot, ICI Pharmaceuticals) on blood loss at surgery for fibroids. Twenty women from the group acted as controls: nine for myomectomy and 11 for hysterectomy. The remaining 22 women received treatment preoperatively in the form of Zoladex® depot 3.6 mg subcutaneously monthly for 4 months. Nine of these 22 women subsequently underwent hysterectomy and 13 underwent myomectomy. Each patient had monthly haemoglobin estimations carried out, and ultrasound scans to assess the size of the uterus. The surgery was carried out by one of two surgeons, in order to standardize the techniques used, and no myomectomy clamps or vasoconstrictive agents were used during any of the surgical procedures. No iron supplements were prescribed to either group of patients, preoperatively.

After routine opening of the abdomen, the swabs used for this part of the procedure were discarded, and the swabs soiled subsequently during the actual myomectomy or hysterectomy were saved until the closure of the peritoneum. The amount of blood absorbed by the swabs during the operation was then measured by the alkaline haematin technique[7]. For this, the swabs were soaked in caustic soda, as was a known volume of venous blood from the patient taken immediately before opening the abdomen. The volume of caustic soda used was noted. From the resulting solutions, the volume of blood (ml) contained in the collected swabs may be calculated using the formula:

$$\frac{\text{OD blood loss} \times \text{volume venous blood}}{\text{OD venous blood}} \times \text{volume NaOH}$$

where OD = optical density. The total amount of blood lost at operation was calculated from the sum of the amount of blood absorbed in the swabs and the amount collected in the suction bottle during the operation.

RESULTS

Uterine size

All patients who had hysterectomy following treatment with goserelin had shrunken fibroids (Figure 1), while those undergoing hysterectomy in the non-treatment control group showed no shrinkage – indeed the fibroids had enlarged significantly in three of the women (Figure 2).

Similarly in the myomectomy group, those treated had fibroids which shrank in the 4-month treatment period preoperatively (Figure 3), while those in the myomectomy control group exhibited no such change in size of their fibroids (Figure 4).

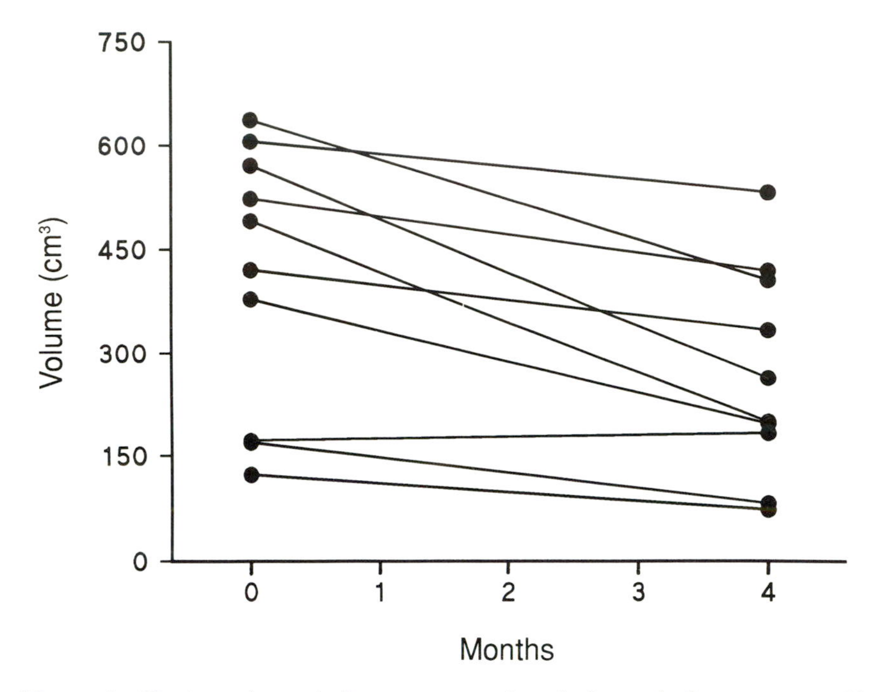

Figure 1 Uterine volumes in hysterectomy patients before and after treatment with goserelin

The shrinkage in size of the fibroids in the treatment groups was so substantial in 9 cases that a transverse lower abdominal incision could be used rather than a lower abdominal midline or right paramedian incision, which would have been mandatory had the patient not undergone pretreatment with goserelin. This was considered by the patients to be a further advantage of the use of goserelin.

Bleeding on treatment

GnRH analogues have been used to treat menorrhagia, albeit temporarily[8]. Women treated with goserelin depot with dysfunctional bleeding had a scanty withdrawal bleed in the first month of therapy and then remained amenorrhoeic until the effect of the final depot wore off, the menses then returning to the former volume[9]. Williams and Shaw

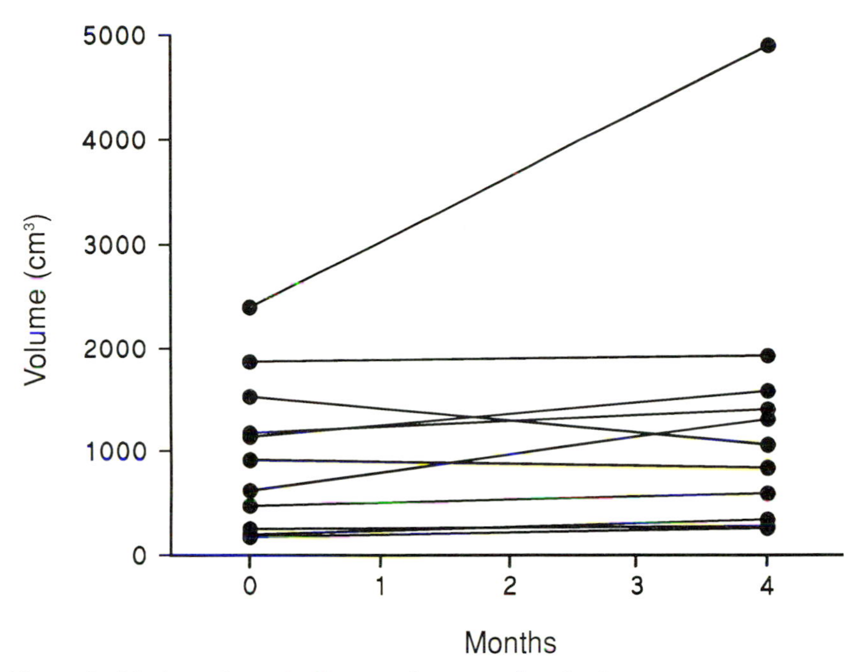

Figure 2 Uterine volumes in the control group undergoing hysterectomy

reported bleeding during treatment with nafarelin, when used to shrink fibroids, and although the blood loss was only subjectively assessed by the patients themselves, the loss was in general lighter although more prolonged in those women that bled on therapy[10].

In our study using goserelin depot to treat fibroids, only eight of the 22 women treated reported bleeding during the treatment period of 4 months, but it was less than the individuals' normal menstrual loss, both on subjective and objective assessment. Figure 5 shows the blood loss in a typical patient who bled during treatment with goserelin prior to undergoing myomectomy, and follows her haemoglobin levels during treatment and in the postoperative period. It can be seen from the graph that the blood loss lessened during therapy, and this was mirrored by a rise in haemoglobin. At surgery, where eight fibroids were removed through three uterine incisions the loss was not excessive, her haemoglobin fell at the time of surgery, and rose without the aid of iron as her menses

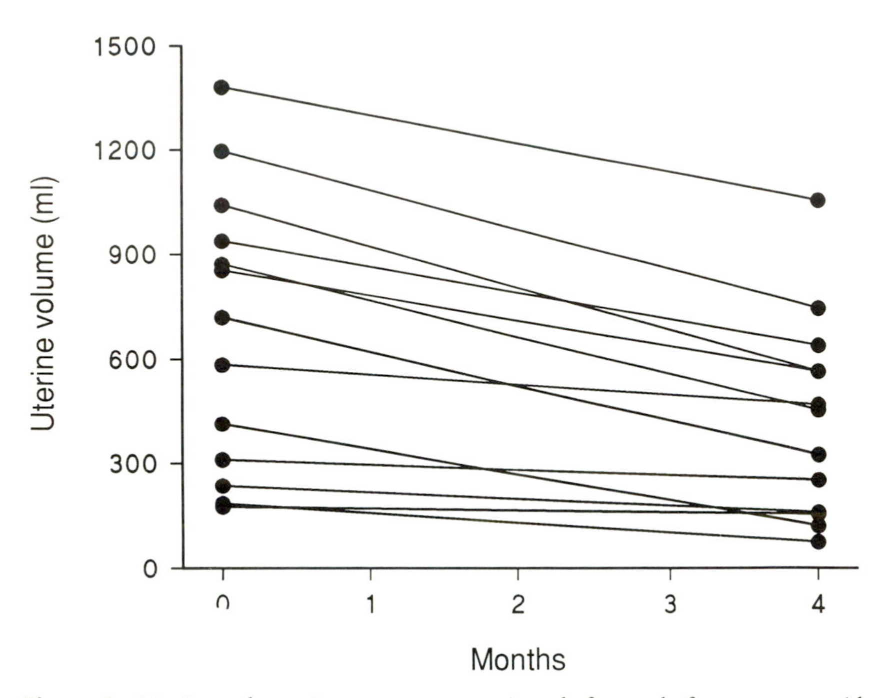

Figure 3 Uterine volumes in myomectomy patients before and after treatment with goserelin

continued in the normal range of loss. This woman remains well some two years after her myomectomy and has not reported any heavy bleeding. This suggests that myomectomy has a beneficial effect on the menstrual blood loss where it is excessive preoperatively, and that the reduction postoperatively is not due to the use of GnRH agonist, since its effect on the menstrual blood loss is only temporary.

The effect of GnRH agonists on haemoglobin

Mean haemoglobin levels in the hysterectomy patients show a higher preoperative level in the treated group compared to the controls (Table 1), while the postoperative levels were similar. The reason for this is not clear since those in the treated group did not lose as much blood peroperatively as those in the control group.

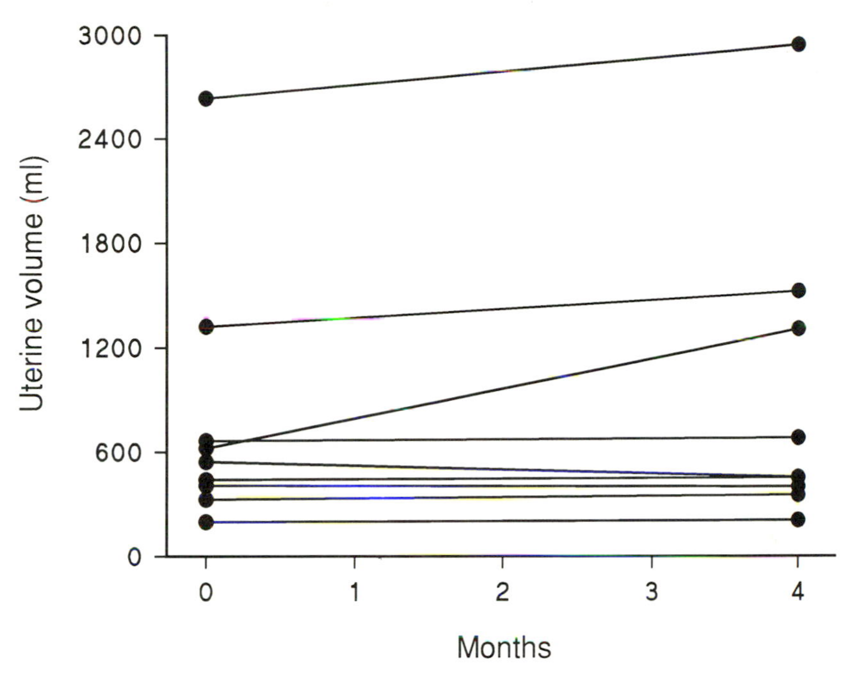

Figure 4 Uterine volumes in the control group undergoing myomectomy

Table 1 Mean haemoglobin levels in patients treated with goserelin prior to surgery for fibroids and in controls

	Haemoglobin levels (g/dl)	
Surgery/period	*Treated*	*Controls*
Hysterectomy		
Time 0	11.9	11.7
Preoperative	13.2	12.3
Postoperative	11.2	11.0
Myomectomy		
Time 0	11.6	11.3
Preoperative	12.5	11.0
Postoperative	11.5	10.4

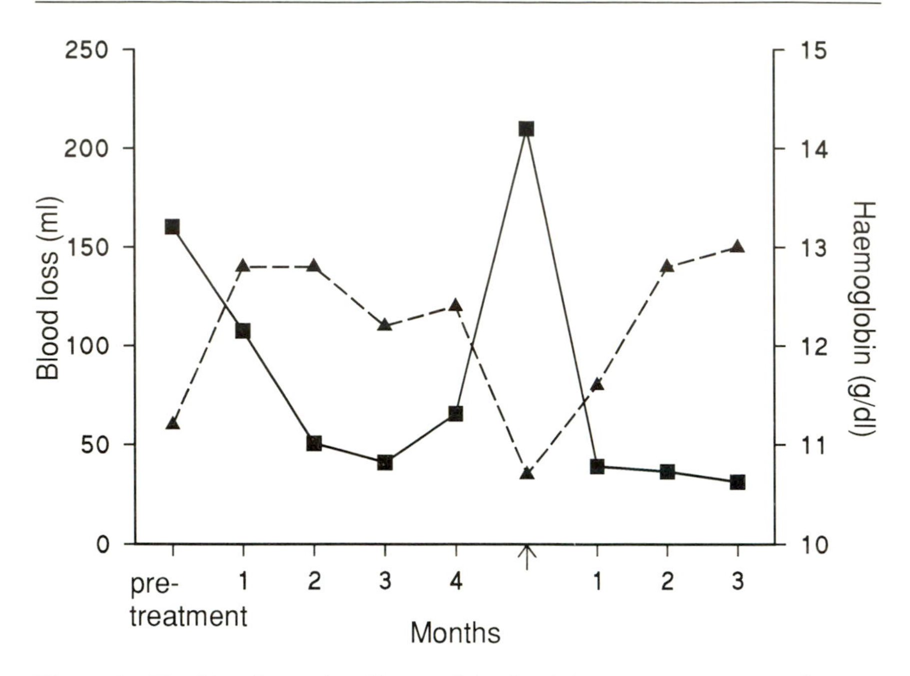

Figure 5 Blood loss (■——■) and haemoglobin levels (▲---▲) in a patient undergoing myomectomy (arrow)

Mean haemoglobin levels in the myomectomy patients show a higher level both pre and postoperatively in the treated group of patients compared with the control group, and this is most likely to be a reflection of the lesser blood loss at surgery in the treated group (Table 1).

Blood loss at surgery

Table 2 illustrates the blood loss at surgery in the treated and untreated groups of both patients undergoing myomectomy and hysterectomy. In both types of surgery, the blood loss was substantially reduced where the patient had been treated preoperatively with goserelin depot. This could be accounted for in the myomectomy group by the number of fibroids removed and the number of incisions being less in the treated group. This was not the case, as can be seen from Table 3. In fact, the maximum number of fibroids removed from a single patient in the treated group was

Table 2 Blood loss at surgery for fibroids, measured objectively using the alkaline haematin technique

	Blood loss (ml)			
	n	*Treated*	*n*	*Controls*
Hysterectomy	9	181.9	11	350.1
Myomectomy	13	304.1	9	502.3

Table 3 Mean peroperative blood loss compared with the number of fibroids removed at myomectomy

	Blood loss (ml)	
Number of fibroids removed	*Treated*	*Controls*
1–2	370	565
3–4	278	960
5–8	310	596
9–13	450	588
> 13	860	—

33, from 8 incisions into the uterus. In short, there was no correlation between the blood loss at surgery and the number of fibroids removed or the number of incisions made into the uterus, suggesting that the GnRH agonist goserelin had a beneficial effect on the amount of blood lost at surgery. It was also interesting to note that the estimated blood loss at the time of surgery showed little or no correlation with the actual amount measured by the alkaline haematin technique, and only gave a rough guide as to whether the blood loss was a normal or excessive amount.

Blood transfusions

Of the 42 women who underwent surgery for their fibroids, 12 received blood transfusions. As expected from the nature of the surgery, the incidence of blood transfusion was higher in those women undergoing myomectomy. Three women in the hysterectomy group required transfusion, and nine in the myomectomy group. The reasons for transfusion are illustrated in Table 4 and 5. In the treated hysterectomy

Table 4 Blood transfusions in hysterectomy patients

	Blood loss (ml)	*Number of units transfused*	*Reason*
Treated group	183	2	Excessive subjective loss
Control group	487	2	Anaemic preoperatively
	177	4	Anaemic preoperatively

Table 5 Blood transfusions in myomectomy patients. All transfusions were administered for subjective excessive blood loss at surgery

	Blood loss (ml)	*Number of units transfused*
Controls	1322	3
	1065	4*
	768	2
	770	2
	628	2
Pretreated group	169	2†
	1070	2
	377	2†
	1130	2
	146	2

* Myomectomy abandoned and patient underwent hysterectomy
† Borderline anaemia preoperatively

group, one patient only received a blood transfusion on the subjective loss at the time of surgery. Subsequently, when the blood loss had been measured objectively, it was found to be only 183 ml, and the patients' postoperative haemoglobin reflected that the transfusion of 2 units of blood had been unnecessary. In the control group for hysterectomy, two patients were transfused preoperatively for persistent anaemia.

In the myomectomy patients, five patients in the treated group and five patients in the control group were transfused peroperatively. Again it can be seen from Table 5 that the blood loss in three of the patients, when measured objectively, did not warrant blood transfusion, whereas in the control group, all the patients transfused required blood transfusion from the objective blood-loss measurement. Indeed, in the control group, one patient bled so substantially that the procedure of myomectomy was abandoned and the patient underwent hysterectomy.

CONCLUSIONS

The mean haemoglobin levels in the two treated groups were higher preoperatively than in the untreated groups without resorting to iron therapy, giving rise to a lower incidence of blood transfusion in the treated groups of patients. Less blood was lost at both hysterectomy and myomectomy at operation in the treated groups of patients.

From this study, it can be seen that there is a lower incidence of blood transfusion in patients who received pretreatment than in those who received no goserelin depot prior to surgery for fibroids. The incidence of blood transfusion was higher in the group who underwent myomectomy, as expected, since there is a greater potential for excessive blood loss during this procedure. The incidence of blood transfusion was particularly low in the group treated with goserelin prior to hysterectomy and slightly lower in the group treated prior to myomectomy.

These factors lead to the conclusion that pretreatment with a GnRH agonist is beneficial to the patients' well-being where surgery for fibroids is indicated. Where small accessible fibroids are present, the use of a GnRH agonist may possibly shrink the fibroids further to such a size that a previously unsuitable endoscopic technique to remove them may then be possible. Certainly in our study the fibroids were often shrunk to such a size that it was possible to remove the uterus or fibroids through a transverse incision as opposed to a vertical incision, which would have been mandatory had the fibroids retained their former size.

REFERENCES

1. Maheux, R., Lemay, A. and Merat, P. (1987). Use of intranasal luteinising hormone-releasing hormone agonist in uterine leiomyomas. *Fertil. Steril.*, **47**, 229–33
2. Lemay, A., Maheux, R., Faure, M., Jean, C. and Fazekas, A. (1984). Reversible hypogonadism induced by a luteinising hormone-releasing hormone (LHRH) agonist (buserelin) as a new therapeutic approach to endometriosis. *Fertil. Steril.*,**41**, 863–71
3. Matta, W.H.M., Stabile, I., Shaw, R. and Campbell, S. (1988). Doppler assessment of uterine blood flow changes in patients with fibroids receiving the gonadotrophin-releasing hormone agonist, buserelin. *Fertil. Steril.*, **49**, 1083–5
4. Matta, W.H.M., Shaw, R.W. and Nye, M. (1989). Long-term follow-up of patients with uterine fibroids after treatment with the LHRH agonist, buserelin. *Br. J. Obstet. Gynaecol.*, **96**, 200–6
5. Stevenson, J., Lees, B., Gardner, R. and Shaw, R.W. (1989). Prolonged effects of an LHRH agonist, goserelin, on the skeleton. Presented at the *Silver Jubilee British Congress of Obstetrics and Gynaecology*, London, July 1989
6. Matta, W., Shaw, R., Hesp, R. and Evans, R. (1988). Reversible trabecular bone density loss following induced hypo-oestrogenism with the LHRH analogue buserelin in premenopausal women. *Clin. Endocrinol.*, **29**, 45–51
7. Hallberg, L. and Nilsson, L. (1961). Determination of menstrual blood loss. *Scand. J. Clin. Lab. Invest.*, **16**, 244–8
8. Shaw, R. and Fraser, H. (1984). Use of superactive luteinising hormone-releasing hormone agonist in the treatment of menorrhagia. *Br. J. Obstet. Gynaecol.*, **91**, 913–16
9. Gardner, R. and Shaw, R.W. (1990). LHRH analogues in the treatment of menorrhagia. In Shaw, R.W. (ed.) *Advances in Reproductive Endocrinology, Vol. 2, Dysfunctional Uterine Bleeding*, pp.149–60. (Carnforth, UK: Parthenon Publishing)
10. Williams, I.A. and Shaw, R.W. (1990). Effect of nafarelin on uterine fibroids measured by ultrasound and magnetic resonance imaging. *Eur. J. Obstet. Gynaecol. Reprod. Biol.*, **34**, 111–17

14

Treatment of fibroids with the combination of the GnRH agonist goserelin (Zoladex®) and hormone replacement therapy

R. Maheux

INTRODUCTION

Gonadotropin-releasing hormone (GnRH) agonists reduce the size of uterine leiomyoma by half and relieve patients of symptoms such as menorrhagia and pelvic pain[1]. They reduce uterine blood flow[2], and increase haemoglobin and haematocrit concentration[3]. Unfortunately, rapid regrowth frequently occurs after therapy is stopped. For pre-menopausal women harbouring a benign pathology such as uterine leiomyoma, long-term treatment with GnRH agonists may represent an alternative to hysterectomy, especially during the years immediately preceding the menopause. However, side-effects such as hot flushes and possible bone-mass reduction have precluded the use of long-term treatment with these agents.

Evidence suggests that severe hypo-oestrogenism is not necessary to shrink uterine leiomyoma and that symptoms may be controlled with minimal incidence of hot flushes or deleterious effects on bone mass. We reported that administration of the GnRH agonist, buserelin, by nasal spray (400 μg, three times a day)[4] is as effective as when the agent is given by subcutaneous injection (500 μg once a day)[1] for the treatment of uterine leiomyoma, although oestradiol levels were significantly less suppressed during treatment and patients had fewer hot flushes. Adjusting the dosage of GnRH agonist in order to conserve some oestrogen stimulation without regrowth of the leiomyoma or recurrence of abnormal bleeding is, however, difficult[5].

The purpose of this study was to evaluate the effects of treatment with a monthly depot formulation of the GnRH agonist, goserelin, in combination with hormone replacement therapy (conjugated oestrogens, 0.3 mg and medroxyprogesterone acetate, 5 mg) in patients with uterine leiomyoma. Parameters studied included volume of uterine leiomyoma, patient symptomatology and bleeding patterns, bone mineral content, and cholesterol fractions.

MATERIALS AND METHODS

Twenty women were referred to our centre for surgery or second opinion about surgery, and were between 39 and 51 years of age (mean and SEM: 45.4 ± 0.79). They were enrolled in this study between May 1987 and June 1990. Four patients were smokers. No patient had a past history of fractures or osteoporosis and all had normal bone densitometry before the study. Ten patients had one leiomyoma, five had 2 tumours, two patients had 3 tumours, and three patients had 4 myomas, respectively. The mean initial volume of the leiomyoma in these patients was 215.8 ± 73 cm^3. Twelve patients complained of menorrhagia (six with associated anaemia) and three of polyuria and nocturia, the remaining patients presenting with pelvic pain and/or pelvic pressure. Inclusion criteria were as follows: age between 39 and 51 years, symptomatic uterine leiomyoma evaluated by gynaecological examination and ultrasound, normal ovulatory cycles (normal basal body temperature chart and serum luteal progesterone > 3 ng/ml), and a normal endometrial biopsy. Exclusion criteria were: menopause (follicle stimulating hormone (FSH) > 40 IU/l), pregnancy or breast feeding, previous hormonal therapy (including oral contraceptives) during the last 6 months, history of thromboembolism, liver or heart disease, body weight more than 2 standard deviations above the expected weight (Metropolitan Life Insurance Table).

Pre-study tests and evaluation included complete medical history, physical examination, FSH, luteinizing hormone (LH), oestradiol, progesterone, pelvic ultrasound, complete haemogram, urinalysis, blood urea nitrogen, creatinine, electrolytes, glycaemia, total proteins, albumin, human chorionic gonadotropin (hCG), cholesterol, high-density lipoprotein cholesterol, triglycerides, and dual-photon bone densitometry of the lumbar spine and the femoral neck.

The GnRH agonist goserelin (Zoladex®, ICI Pharma, Mississauga, Ontario, Canada), in the form of a biodegradable cylindrical depot containing 3.6 mg of the compound, was injected subcutaneously every 28 days in the lower anterior abdominal wall using a prepacked syringe. Local anaesthesia was used initially in one patient. Treatment was started on days 2–5 of the cycle and continued for 12 months. After the first 3 months of goserelin administration, low-dose hormonal replacement therapy was added to the treatment regimen. The first 10 patients (Group A) received conjugated equine oestrogens 0.3 mg (Premarin®, Ayerst Laboratories, Montreal, P.Q., Canada) on days 1–25 of each cycle, and medroxyprogesterone acetate 5 mg (Provera®, Upjohn Canada, Mississauga, Ontario, Canada) on days 16–25. The remaining 10 patients (Group B) received the same medications continuously from the first day of the third month to the last day of the twelfth month.

Patients' clinical symptoms were reviewed and pelvic ultrasound and serum oestradiol determinations were performed at the time of each monthly goserelin depot injection. All patients were advised to take 1.5 g of calcium in their daily diet. A complete physical examination and the laboratory tests were performed every 3 months and at the 3-month follow-up visit. Bone densitometry assessments were repeated after 6 and 12 months of therapy and at the 3-month follow-up visit. Endometrial biopsy was repeated only at the end of the therapy.

Serum oestradiol was measured by a solid-phase ^{125}I-radioimmunoassay using an antibody-coated tube (Diagnostic Products Corporation, Los Angeles, USA). The assay sensitivity was 20–40 pmol/l. The intra- and interassay variations at 180 pmol/l were 7% and 8.1%, respectively. Serum triglycerides and total cholesterol were measured by enzymatic methods on a Hitachi 705 autoanalyser using Boehringer Mannheim reagents. High-density lipoprotein cholesterol was determined using the heparin-$MnCl_2$ precipitation method[6].

Ultrasound determinations of leiomyoma volume were performed with an Aloka SSD 280 (Aloka Company Ltd, Tokyo, Japan) with a 3.5 MHz transducer. Leiomyoma volume was calculated using the formula $4/\pi r^3$. The diagnosis of uterine leiomyoma by ultrasonography has been validated in a previous study[7]. For standardization of calculation, when more than one leiomyoma was identified during treatment, their volumes were added together.

Bone densitometry was performed using a biphotonic densitometer (Lunar Radiation Corporation, Madison, Wisconsin, USA) with a precision of 4%. Both the lumbar spine and femoral neck regions were evaluated.

Data were computerized and analyzed using the paired Student's *t*-test with comparisons of mean values between month zero (pretreatment) and subsequent months, with 0.05 as the level of significance. If a patient withdrew from the study, the paired Student's *t*-test was calculated on the remaining patients.

RESULTS

Endocrine response

As shown in Figure 1, mean oestradiol levels decreased significantly ($p < 0.001$) from 284.7 ± 62.9 pmol/l before the study to 31.8 ± 5.3 pmol/l after 3 months of treatment. With the addition of hormonal replacement therapy, mean oestradiol levels (at the time of monthly goserelin depot injection) oscillated between 93.6 ± 23.4 and 157.8 ± 24.7 pmol/l, then rapidly returned to pre-study levels after treatment (307.3 ± 63.4 pmol/l after 3 months of follow-up).

Uterine volume

The volume of uterine leiomyoma significantly decreased ($p < 0.001$) during the first 3 months compared to the initial volume (100%). The mean volume of the leiomyoma in the patients was $46.5 \pm 4.5\%$ after 3 months of treatment. Mean tumour volume did not change significantly with the addition of oestrogen and progestin at month 4, varying between $46.5 \pm 6.2\%$ and $71.7 \pm 16\%$ of the initial volume during the final 9-month treatment period. After 3 months of follow-up, the mean volume of leiomyoma had increased to pre-study values (mean = $108.7 \pm 16.8\%$; a difference from the mean versus pre-study tumour volume which was

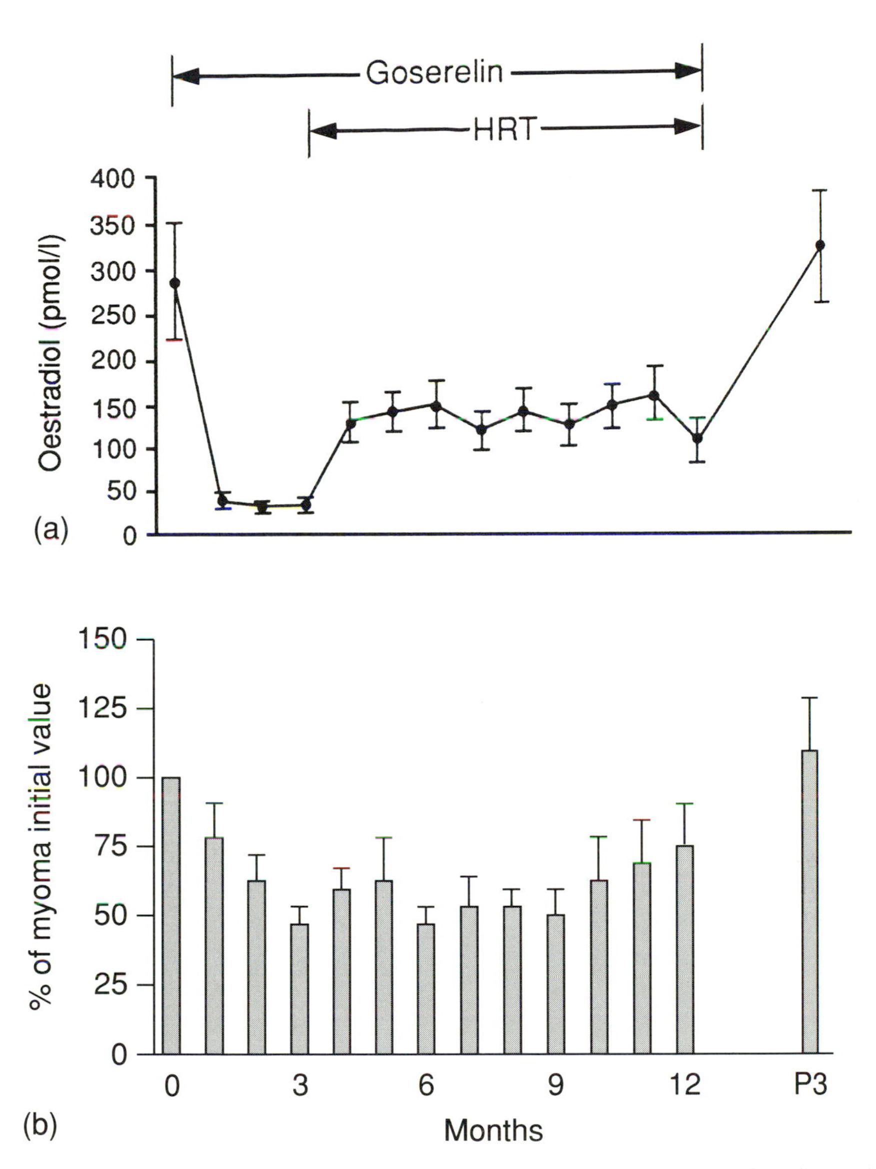

Figure 1 (a) Mean (± SEM, indicated by bars) serum oestradiol levels and (b) volume of uterine leiomyoma during treatment and follow-up

not significant) and normal menses rapidly returned. The relative re-increase in the mean volume of leiomyoma during the last 3 months of treatment was related to one patient (case 1, Group B) in whom the leiomyoma regrew progressively from 75% of the initial volume at month 6 to 301% at month 12; after 3 months of follow-up, the leiomyoma had decreased to 91% of the initial volume in this subject.

Bleeding pattern, endometrial biopsy and haemoglobin

Figures 2 and 3 illustrate the bleeding pattern reported during therapy with cyclic (Group A) and continuous (Group B) hormone replacement therapy respectively. Although a clear improvement over the pre-study bleeding pattern was observed in both treatment groups, much better control of bleeding was observed following the utilization of continuous vs. cyclic hormone replacement therapy. Endometrial biopsies, which were compatible with normal luteal phase before the study, were compatible with atrophic changes or slight proliferative endometrium at the end of the study. In the five patients who presented with low haemoglobin levels before the study, mean serum haemoglobin levels increased during treatment from 10.5 ± 1.1 g/l at the initiation of treatment to 12.6 ± 0.8 g/l at month 12.

Clinical side-effects

All patients experienced hot flushes. These hot flushes, which usually started during the second month of goserelin therapy, were severe in six patients during the third month of therapy. With the addition of hormone replacement therapy, they progressively disappeared in most patients. Control of hot flushes was superior in patients receiving continuous (Group B), as opposed to cyclic hormone replacement therapy (Group A). The pelvic pain and pelvic pressure present before the start of therapy almost completely disappeared during treatment.

Two patients did not complete the study. Patient number 7 stopped treatment at month 4 because of headaches, insomnia and recurrence of heavy bleeding with hormone replacement therapy. Patient number 10 stopped treatment at the tenth visit because of hot flushes.

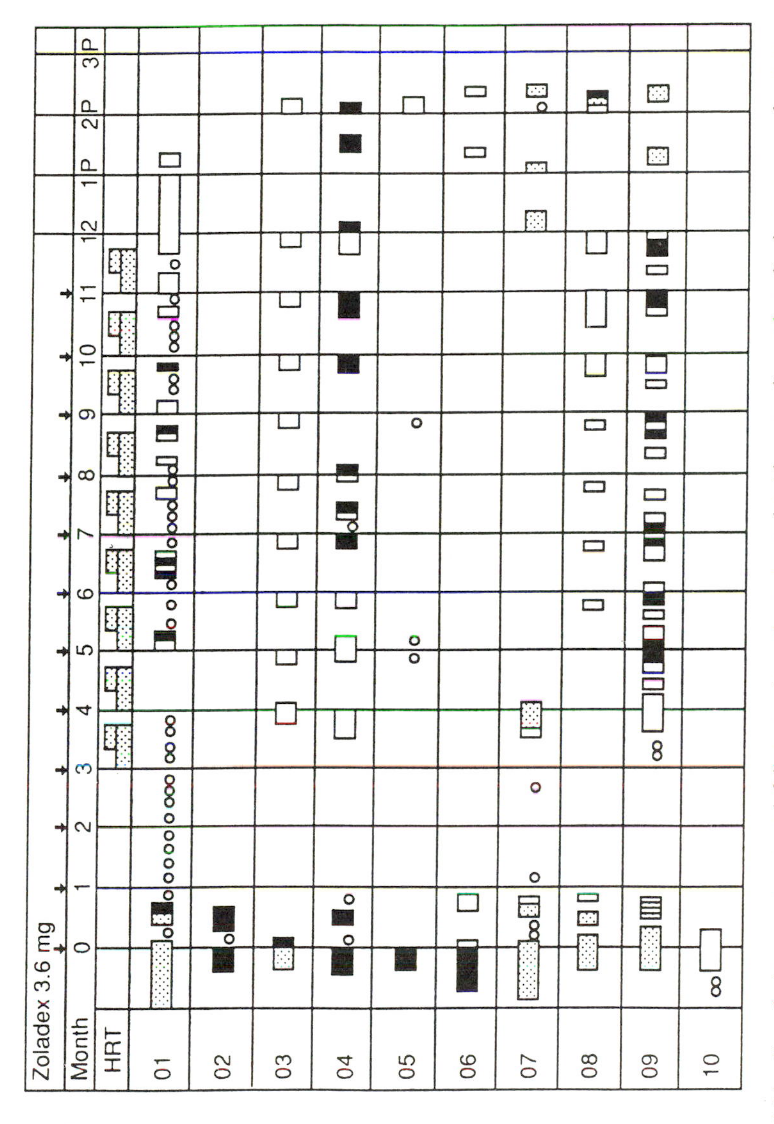

Figure 2 Vaginal bleeding during treatment and follow-up in patients treated with goserelin and cyclic hormone replacement therapy (HRT). Abscissae = month of treatment; ordinates = patient number

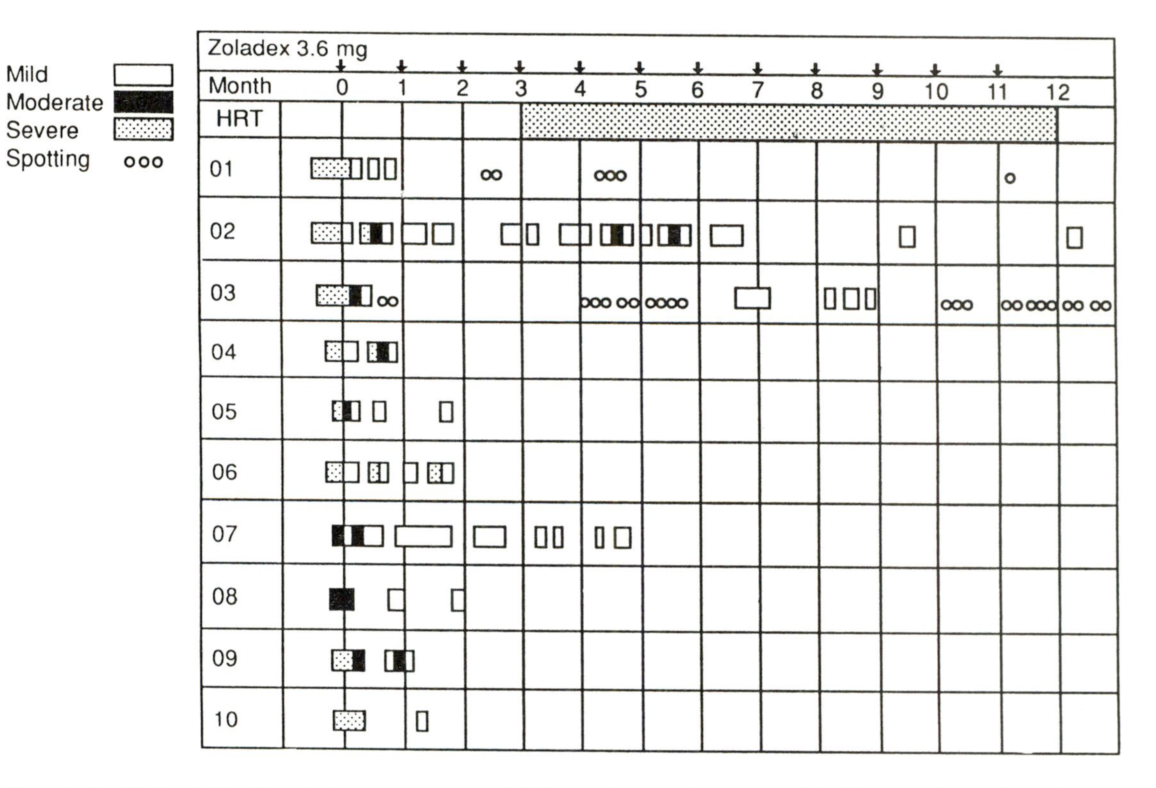

Figure 3 Vaginal bleeding during treatment and follow-up in patients treated with goserelin and continuous hormone replacement therapy (HRT). Abscissae = month of treatment; ordinates = patient number

Ovulation, as assessed by basal body temperature, occurred an average 86.6 ± 9.1 days after the last injection of goserelin. No other side-effects were reported except occasional headaches.

Bone density

As shown in Table 1, bone density decreased during the first 6 months of treatment. The difference from baseline was statistically significant ($p < 0.05$) at months 6 and 12 for L2–L4. Three months after cessation of therapy, L2–L4 bone density was no different from pretreatment values. No statistically significant difference in bone density at the femoral neck was observed either during or after treatment. There was no correlation between initial bone density and variation observed with treatment. No significant difference in terms of effects on bone density was observed between the two treatment groups.

Table 1 Bone density of the lumbar spine (L2–L4) and the femoral neck during treatment and follow-up

	Number of patients	*Mean (± SEM) bone density* (g/cm^2)	
		L2–L4	*Femoral neck*
Pre-study	20	1.05 ± 0.04	0.82 ± 0.03
6 months	19	0.98 ± 0.05*	0.80 ± 0.03
12 months	17	1.00 ± 0.05*	0.71 ± 0.07
+3 months	18	1.03 ± 0.05	0.81 ± 0.03

*$p < 0.05$

Lipid profile and other biological parameters

Table 2 shows the patients' lipid profiles during treatment and follow-up. Mean cholesterol levels slightly, but significantly, increased during treatment. High-density lipoprotein cholesterol concentrations also increased during treatment, reaching significance only at month 9. There

Table 2 Serum triglycerides, cholesterol, high-density lipoprotein cholesterol level, cholesterol/high-density lipoprotein cholesterol ratio during treatment and follow-up. All figures are means ± SEM, mmol/l

Months	*Number of patients*	*Triglycerides*	*Cholesterol*	*High-density lipoprotein cholesterol*	*Cholesterol/high-density lipoprotein cholesterol*
0	20	1.13 ± 0.13	4.79 ± 0.15	1.56 ± 0.09	3.23 ± 0.18
3	20	1.21 ± 0.12	5.22 ± 0.21**	1.65 ± 0.01	3.24 ± 0.17
6	19	1.31 ± 0.11	5.14 ± 0.18**	1.59 ± 0.09	3.36 ± 0.16
9	19	1.25 ± 0.12	5.13 ± 0.18*	1.59 ± 0.08*	3.33 ± 0.18
12	18	1.34 ± 0.11	5.08 ± 0.16	1.56 ± 0.07	3.39 ± 0.19

*$p < 0.05$
**$p < 0.01$

was no significant increase in the atherogenic index (cholesterol/high-density lipoprotein cholesterol ratio). Plasma triglyceride concentrations did not change significantly during treatment. All the other biological parameters investigated were within the normal range before, during, and after the treatment period and did not change significantly during the study period. No significant difference in lipid or other biological parameters was observed between the two treatment groups.

DISCUSSION

The mean volume of uterine leiomyoma was reduced by half after 3 months of treatment with goserelin, a monthly subcutaneous depot GnRH agonist. Addition of low-dose conjugated equine oestrogens and medroxyprogesterone acetate to goserelin for 9 months did not result in a significant increase in leiomyoma volume or symptomatology and reduced the incidence of side-effects reported with goserelin alone. These results confirm our initial findings which showed shrinkage of uterine leiomyoma during incomplete oestrogen suppression by an intranasal GnRH-agonist[4]. The rapid and complete oestradiol suppression achieved with the GnRH agonist implant provides an opportunity to use hormone replacement therapy for maintaining steroid at stable levels during treatment.

Better control of vaginal bleeding and hot flushes was observed during the last 9 months of the study with the addition of continuous hormone replacement therapy compared with the cyclic regimen. It is therefore our opinion that when hormone replacement therapy is used in conjunction with GnRH agonist treatment, a continuous regimen is preferable to a cyclic one.

Monitoring of patients' plasma lipid profiles during treatment did not reveal any deleterious effect on the lipid profile. The observed increase in cholesterol levels during treatment, although significant, was small. There was also a small increase in high-density lipoprotein cholesterol concentrations; however, there was no significant change in the atherogenic index. In this study, the administration of 0.3 mg of conjugated oestrogens and 5 mg of medroxyprogesterone acetate was associated with a significant demineralization of the trabecular bone of the lumbar vertebrae during the first 6 months of treatment. There was a small re-increase in bone density at month 12, and 3 months after cessation of the treatment, bone density was back to pre-study values.

The utilization of a higher dosage of hormone replacement therapy such as 0.625 mg of conjugated equine oestrogens and 10 mg of medroxyprogesterone acetate[8] may offer better protection against bone loss. However, some patients (such as patient number 1 in treatment Group B) may be more sensitive than others when hormone replacement therapy is added to GnRH agonist treatment; a higher dosage may not, therefore, be well tolerated by all patients. In addition, higher dosage of hormone replacement therapy is often associated with regular withdrawal bleeding, a major problem for compliance in menopausal women receiving such therapy; a continuous regimen may help to solve this problem.

The addition of hormone replacement therapy allows longer-term GnRH agonist treatment and the possibility, if necessary, of administering this regimen more than once. The utilization of a depot formulation of GnRH agonist makes treatment more practical for the patient; longer-term depot formulations (3 months) may represent a further improvement if they become available. As most women who are older than 40 years having a hysterectomy will also have a bilateral salpingo-oopherectomy and be placed on hormone replacement therapy, depot GnRH agonist treatment combined with such therapy may offer a valid alternative to hysterectomy during the immediate years preceding the menopause, when the pathology involved is not malignant or pre-malignant. GnRH agonist therapy is, however, expensive and its safety on long-term usage, even with the addition of hormone replacement therapy, has not yet been demonstrated in large-scale studies. These preliminary results are, however, encouraging and should lead us to larger prospective randomized trials with untreated control groups.

REFERENCES

1. Maheux, R., Gilloteau, C., Lemay, A., Bastide, A. and Fazekas, A.T. (1985). Luteinizing hormone-releasing hormone agonist and uterine leiomyoma: a pilot study. *Am. J. Obstet. Gynecol.*, **152**, 1034–8
2. Matta, W.H.M., Stabile, I., Shaw, R.W. and Campbell, S. (1988). Doppler assessment of uterine blood flow changes in patients with fibroids receiving the gonadotrophin-releasing hormone agonist, buserelin. *Fertil. Steril.*, **49**, 1083–5
3. West, C.P., Williamson, J., Lumsden, M.A., Baird, D.T. and Lawson, S. (1987). Shrinkage of uterine fibroids during therapy with goserelin (Zoladex): a luteinizing hormone-releasing hormone agonist administered as a monthly subcutaneous depot. *Fertil. Steril.*, **48**, 45–51
4. Maheux, R., Lemay, A. and Merat, P. (1987). Use of intranasal luteinizing hormone-releasing hormone agonist in uterine leiomyomas. *Fertil. Steril.*, **47**, 229–33
5. Maheux, R. (1986). LH-RH agonists – How useful against uterine leiomyomas? *Contemp. Obstet. Gynecol.*, **28**, 66–77
6. Warnick, G.R. and Albers, J.J.A. (1978). A comprehensive evaluation of heparin-manganese precipitation procedure for estimating high density lipoprotein cholesterol. *J. Lipid Res.*, **19**, 65–76
7. Maheux, R., Marcoux, S., Guilloteaa-Paudonson, C., Paquet, N. and Jean, C. (1987). Validity of gynecologic exam and pelvic ultrasound in the diagnosis of leiomyomata uteri. *Infertility*, **10**, 15–21
8. Friedman, A.J., Benacerras, B., Harrison-Atlas, D., Gleason, R., Barbieri, R.L. and Schiff, I. (1989). A randomised, placebo-controlled, double-blind study evaluating the efficacy of leuprolide acetate depot in the treatment of uterine leiomyomata. *Fertil. Steril.*, **51**, 251–6

Index

BRITISH COLUMBIA CANCER AGENCY
LIBRARY
600 WEST 10th AVE.
VANCOUVER, B.C. CANADA
V5Z 4E6